THE ENGLISH DOCTOR

THE ENGLISH DOCTOR

A Medical Journey

Dr Richard Sloan

To order additional copies of this book, contact:
Xlibris Corporation
0-800-644-6988
www.Xlibrispublishing.co.uk
Orders@Xlibrispublishing.co.uk
304037

CONTENTS

This book is dedicated to all those who have enabled me to travel on a marvellous medical journey. They include my parents, who supported my education and the many colleagues for and with whom I have worked. I also dedicate this book to the thousands of patients I have met and tried to help. Above all, I dedicate this book to my wife, Kathleen Sloan, who is my rock.

INTRODUCTION

I have had an unusual career as a scientist, undergraduate lecturer, educationalist, mentor, and general medical practitioner (GP).

The intention of this book is to capture the essence of medical research and medical practice during the second half of the twentieth century and the start of the twenty-first. I have focussed on what happens behind the scenes as a student, house officer, undergraduate lecturer, research worker, GP, postgraduate educator, and NHS manager. I am sure the average UK patient, and indeed many health-care workers, including doctors, has no idea of what went on behind the scenes. Those doctors who were GP trainees in Yorkshire as well as those who were developed as trainers were so lucky to have some of the most interesting and skilled teachers in the UK.

This book is about my experiences, views, and the colleagues who have contributed to the direction of my medical journey. After the first chapter about my early life, I have purposely not written much about my personal life as the book is not intended to be an autobiography in the purest sense. I have included anecdotes and mentioned many people. This is because I do not want this book to be a text book. I apologise to those whom I have omitted to mention and who have contributed to my journey. I also apologise for not explaining fully some of the medical terminology used.

The British Medical Association has published guidelines for the medical profession when writing about patients. Written consent has been obtained for any named patients and an attempt has been made to anonymise the cases that have been described.

I am grateful to Dr Liz Moulton for feeding back to me on the final manuscript and advising me about any possible breaches of confidentiality and any other ethical matters.

Soon after I started writing, Dr Maggie Eisner and Prof. John Lord kindly read the first draft of Chapter 2 and gave me useful feedback.

I am most grateful to my wife, Kathleen, who gave me feedback after each chapter.

My godson, Nick Earls, a successful novelist in Australia, gave me valuable advice on a chapter in the very early stages of writing this book.

My good friend and colleague Grahame Smith gave me useful feedback on the chapter that covered our time together as preclinical medical students, Chapter 2.

Brian Lewis, an artist and writer, gave me valuable advice about publishing.

The last chapter involved talking to many people about their work. They gave up their valuable time freely, and I am most grateful for that.

Prof. Christopher Dean, professor of Anatomy at University College, London, kindly showed me around his department in March 2012 and introduced me to Daniel Wornham, a third-year iB.Sc. student. I am grateful to Daniel for informing me about the preclinical and B.Sc. courses as they were in 2012. Prof. Dean kindly supplied me with the photograph of J Z Young

I am grateful to the dean of research at the Barts and the London School of Medicine and Dentistry, Prof. Thomas MacDonald, for meeting me. He showed me the state-of-the-art research facilities and explained the situation with Ph.D. students and academic teaching. Prof.

Mike Roberts, dean for students, arranged for me to meet three junior doctors working at The Royal London Hospital.

Drs Emile Khan, Natasha Atchamah, and Viyaasan Mahalingasivan told me about clinical medical students and work as foundation year-one doctors.

Thanks to Carol Ward (practice administrator Roehampton Surgery) and Sue Careswell (Leckhampton Surgery, Cheltenham) for talking to me on the telephone and telling me how these practice have developed since I worked there.

I am grateful to Anthony Nicholas (events manager), Linda Reynolds (quality outcome framework lead), Karen Tooley (performance improvement manager), Monica Smith (partner, Tieve Tara Medical Centre), Alison Evans (Wakefield District appraisal lead, NHS Calderdale, Kirklees, and Wakefield District), Adrian Dunbar (associate postgraduate dean, Yorkshire and the Humber Deanery), and David Brown (programme director, West Riding General Practice Specialty Training Programme) for meeting me in 2012 and informing me about their areas of work.

Thanks to the following at Xlibris who have supported me with the writing and publication of this book: Sophia Blake, publishing consultant, Naomi Orleans, author services representative, Chris Lovedice, author consultant and James Calonia, manuscript series representative.

The royalties from this book will be donated to charity.

CHAPTER 1

MY EARLY LIFE

'My Early Life' was the title of an autobiography written by Winston Churchill about his youth. It was one of the set books I read for my O-level English literature examination. In this chapter, I hope to paint a picture of what life was like in a GP's household as I was growing up. There will also be some anecdotes I heard from my father about his work from 1923.

Both my parents were GPs. I was born in 1945. My mother was a private patient in Leeds for my birth. After I was born, she had trouble sleeping. She was given a drug called chloral hydrate. In those days that drug was usually administered in liquid form and had a particular taste. My mother must have taken chloral hydrate previously because immediately after she had swallowed it, she told the nurse that she had been given the wrong dose. It tasted too strong. She had been given ten times the standard dose. My mother had to have a stomach washout. My father was so happy that he did not complain as would have happened now. Instead he filled a cylindrical empty Elastoplast tin with five-pound notes and gave it to the consultant in charge of my delivery.

My mother had three weeks off work before starting work as a full-time GP again. They decided to employ a live-in nanny. She was called Mrs Price. I called her Ninnie. She was over seventy years old, rather overweight, and had osteoarthritis. My father thought that she would be with us for about ten years. How wrong he was! I came back from university to celebrate her ninetieth birthday. She was still living in our house at that time, and my mother took her breakfast in bed. Her arthritis was such that she had to come downstairs backwards. She had her own sitting room and television downstairs. She often was the person who took the messages for the practice when my parents were out. At that time, the surgery was shut each afternoon until the evening surgery started. I got great pleasure from going upstairs and tinkling the telephone bell, then listening to her rushing to the phone to find there was no one there. Each Sunday my parents paid for a 'taxi' to take Mrs Price to visit her daughter Maud for lunch. The 'taxi' was a hearse driven by the local undertaker, Norman Dean.

My father was the first Dr Sloan, and there followed another seventeen of us.

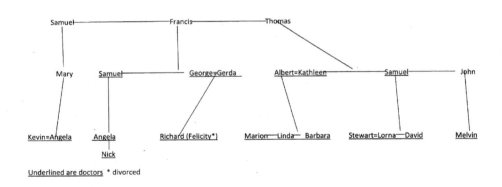

My father, George, went to Queens University, Belfast, to study. As part of his medical studies, he lived in Dublin to learn about obstetrics and for that he was awarded the degree of BAO—Bachelor of the Art of Obstetrics. I think this is a wonderfully sounding degree. Medicine really is an art. There was no such thing as biochemistry when he was at medical school. After he qualified, he worked briefly as a surgeon in Blackburn, Lancashire. He started work as a GP in Halifax, which has some very steep hills up which he sometimes had to reverse his Model T Ford car. The forward gears were not low enough for steep hills.

He went into partnership in 1923 with a fellow Northern Irishman, Dr Gilfillan. Their practice was in Castleford, West Yorkshire. The partnership went wrong and they split up, with Dr Gilfillan taking the more populated Castleford and my father a suburb of Castleford, Airedale. A line was drawn on a map dividing the town into two. They agreed not to treat patients in each other's half. Dr Gilfillan's half had all the prosperous households while the poorer families lived in Airedale. They did not speak to one another for years. In the 1960s, my father and Dr Gilfillan buried the hatchet and made friends again.

There was very little money around in Airedale to pay the GP in the two decades before the Second World War. My father employed a collector called Mr Firth. He had great difficulty getting money from patients. The Great Depression was from 1929 to about 1940, and things were really hard for my father, his first wife, and three children. I think they were relatively poor. That marriage failed and there was a divorce. I had three half-siblings—Francis (Frank), Dorothy (Dot), and Geraldine (Gerry). Dot married Derek, a teacher, and they had three girls—Susan, Carol, and Helen. They came and stayed a lot. In later life, Dorothy had severe Alzheimer's disease, which was terrible to witness. Gerry married Johnny and they had four children—Michael, Andrew, Elizabeth, and David. They are not that much younger than me. Johnny, his father, and sister built up a chain of television shops in Glasgow, which were sold to the Rank Organisation for a large amount of money. Out of the blue, Johnny gave my father the money to buy the car of his dreams—a Jaguar 2. 4 saloon.

Frank lived at home with us for a short time, and we all went on a couple of holidays together. He joined the merchant navy and was on a cargo boat for eighteen months without returning to the UK. On his first day on the boat, the captain assembled the crew and asked, 'Has anyone got a relative who is a doctor?' Frank told him that his father was a GP, and from that point onwards, Frank was the 'ship's doctor'. My father bought a globe of the world to follow Frank's voyages. Frank married Florence, and they adopted two children—Christopher and Mary. Frank and Florence settled in Northern Ireland eventually. Florence is the black sheep of the family. She was thrown out of medical school! She received an MBE for services to young people. Frank became a first radio officer for the Peninsular and Orient line working first on cruise ships, then oil tankers.

Of Frank's generation, only Florence is alive at the time of writing.

My father had a great sense of humour and was always telling jokes and laughing. He smoked Player's cigarettes and was a chain smoker. (My mother gave up smoking forty Player's Weights a day four weeks before I was born.) The waiting room, until I came back to Castleford in 1978, had benches that seated about five adults. On the back of each bench was affixed an ashtray. There was a notice in the waiting room 'No Smoking'. A patient wrote on the notice, 'Why have ashtrays?' My father wrote underneath, 'Because I smoke myself'. Most of his life he felt he had to take the drug chloral hydrate to help him sleep. He once went to a GP about his insomnia and was advised to have a bottle of Guinness at bedtime. My teetotaller father bought a crate of Guinness and put it under the bed. He gave up the Guinness after a short while as it resulted in his having to wake up to go to the lavatory in the middle of the night. The chloral hydrate came in crystal form, which he weighed out on some accurate scales that were in their bedroom. The crystals were then dissolved in water.

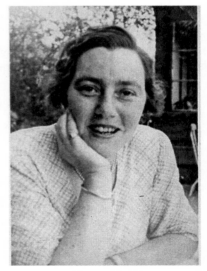

My mother was born in Berlin and was from a very wealthy family. Her father, Richard Leopold Friedman, was a businessman with interests both in Germany and in the United Kingdom. I was called after him. He and my

My mother

grandmother, Lilly, became naturalised British in 1933. They lived in London from that time.

My mother, Gerda Laura Clara Alice, hung on in Berlin until 1938 to fully qualify as a doctor with an MD. The British government interned her bother Herbert and his wife Sania on the Isle of White for the duration of the war. The government ruled that German doctors should take a final examination again. She passed the conjoint examination in Edinburgh (Member of the Royal College of Surgeons, MRCS, and Licentiate of the Royal College of Physicians, LRCP). Shortly after that, the government announced that retaking the finals examination was not required. My mother applied for hundreds of GP jobs. Who on earth was going to take on a German in the middle of the Second World War! In the early 1940s, my father was advertising for an assistant. My mother was an applicant, and he decided to see her. He was not yet divorced, but he said, 'I only hope she is not good looking'.

She got the job and they fell in love. They married on the 30 November 1944, and I was born on 26 November 1945. My mother was placed under a curfew during the war. She was not allowed out after dark. A policeman visited every evening to check she was in, and they had a cup of tea together. My mother thought that the curfew was a great luxury—a GP not allowed to do any night visits!

My mother doted on me. She was a very loving person and spoilt me until the day she died. She had a significant German accent, but her command of the English language was very good. I had a very happy childhood indeed. She read widely and liked a flutter on the horses. She was a good horse rider in her youth. She and my father laughed a lot, and it was obvious to me that they were very much in love. We went on great holidays, and when I reached the age of about seven, the holidays alternated between Lake Tegernsee in Bavaria and a cruise. On the German holiday, we met with her brother, Herbert, and his Russian wife, Sania. They lived in Munich. My mother made sure my father and I were introduced to the theatre and the arts. She took my father to hear Richard Tauber (the German tenor) sing at the Grand

Theatre, Leeds. After the performance, to my father's delight, they went backstage and she introduced him to Tauber. Richard Tauber had been a friend of my grandfather in Berlin. She had not done much cooking up to the time she married. She introduced us to all kinds of food such as the classic German recipe for a beef dish, Esterhazy Rostbraten. She made her own yogurt at a time when no one had heard of yogurt. She was one of the first women in Castleford to wear trousers. My German grandparents moved from London to an apartment in Harrogate during the war, so they were only about 25 miles from us. They stored their valuable art and antiques in two places—London and Berlin. The articles were uninsured. The Germans bombed and destroyed the storage place in London and the British, the one in Berlin.

My father's housekeeper, Mrs Hannah McGrath, gave evidence for him in the divorce court. She was a devout Catholic and was excommunicated by the Roman Catholic Church for doing that.

Our family had a very close relationship with the McGraths as they looked after my father's children when his marriage was in a poor state. Hannah had two daughters, Maureen and Paddy, and one son, Harry. Harry was a prisoner of war in Germany and died from tuberculosis in the early 1960s. I think it demonstrates a great strength of character that Harry got on so well with my German mother. Harry used to chauffeur occasionally for my parents. Maureen's husband, Bert, washed the cars each week. Maureen has been our housekeeper from 1978 to the time of writing in 2011. Maureen had a reserved occupation in the Second World War. A reserved occupation was considered so important that the employee was not expected to do any form of military service, including the women's land army. Maureen's job in that war was to light and tend to the coal fire in the waiting room of the surgery. In 2003, when our huge new medical centre was completed, I asked Maureen to jointly open it with our MP, The Rt Hon Yvette Cooper. There is a plaque in the waiting room with both their names.

Being the only son of parents both of whom were GPs meant I had a thoroughly middle-class and privileged upbringing. I have mentioned that we had a housekeeper, driver, and car washer. We also had a gardener. The gardeners were usually patients who were unable to work or were retired. I remember when I was about five years of age, Mr Siddens was the gardener. He had Parkinson's disease, a feature of which is a tremor, particularly affecting the hands. I remember the strange feeling of a shaky hand patting my head. He made a huge wooden train for me. Another gardener had a severe mental health problem.

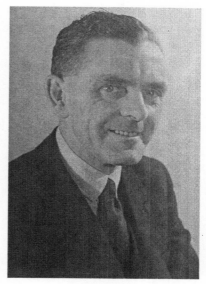

My Father

Tieve Tara was the name of the house and surgery. It was built in 1923 for my father by Fryston Colliery as he was the colliery doctor. Tieve Tara is Gaelic and means the house on the hill.

Fryston is a suburb of Castleford and is a mining village. Fryston is about five minutes' walk from the house. He rented Tieve Tara at first but then bought after a couple of years. He paid £2,000. It was a large five-bedroomed house semi-detached to a small surgery. The house was approached by a private road along which were four other houses all related to the coal mine. Going up the drive, the first house was the manager of the coal mine. It had a tennis court and beautifully maintained garden. The gardeners were miners who also maintained the driveway. The next house was, in the early nineteenth century, a lodge at the gateway to Lord Houghton's estate. (Lord Houghton proposed marriage to Florence Nightingale and was refused.) When I was a child, this house was inhabited by the colliery bookkeeper/accounts manager. Then one comes to Tieve Tara. The next two houses (semi-detached) were for undermanagers of the coal mine. The manager of Fryston Colliery in the 1950s was Mr Jim Bullock, who became quite famous writing a book about coal mining.[1] He always had a huge bonfire on the

---

[1] Jim Bullock. 1972. *Them and Us*. Souvenir Press: London.

5th of November. The wood for that fire was brought up from the pit by miners. One of the undermanagers was Sid Oates. His wife Margaret is ninety-two at the time of writing and my wife and I remain close friends with one of their children, Jennifer. One evening I went around and they were all in tears except for Sid, who was reading the beano comic. Jennifer had sat on the budgerigar, which unfortunately died. The Oates family are good Catholics, and Joey the budgie was given a decent burial. After Jim Bullock retired, the Oates continued with the 5 November bonfire made of wooden pit props. The bonfire was built by coal miners from Fryston Colliery.

Tieve Tara Surgery could be accessed by a rough track from a street called Park Dale. This was a street of mostly nice council houses and was the street where the McGraths lived. I made friends with Norman Wilson and Frank Ward, who lived there. We and John Oates (Jennifer's brother) spent a lot of time playing together. However, I was not allowed to go to Fryston as my parents regarded that place as too rough for me.

As a child and teenager, I was immersed in general practice, which has changed out of all recognition over the past sixty years. In the 1920s and 1930s, my father performed post-mortems, sometimes on his own patients. There was always a policeman in attendance. Not only was my father hard up in the Great Depression, so were the patients, as I have indicated. Some could not afford the vet or dentist. My father extracted teeth and put dogs down during that time.

Until the advent of the health service, the practice dispensed medicines and ointments. The labels for the bottles were handwritten. My mother always maintained that the medicines worked better if my father's handwriting was on the label rather than hers. This is an interesting example of the power of the personality and approach of the doctor on the patient.

In 1948, the National Health Service was born. Patients had to register with a GP. My parent's kindness to patients and good bedside manners paid off. There was a queue stretching far into Park Dale of patients wishing to register. In the mid-1950s, a huge council housing estate was built near the house and surgery and more patients joined. The practice grew to 10,000 patients and my parents took on a partner, Dr Andrew Smith.

Dr Smith had no children. He raced greyhounds. I liked him very much. He had a great reputation looking after children. He was a Scotsman, and on one New Year's Eve, he knocked on our front door. He was first footing. This is a Scottish tradition where the visitor arrives at midnight and is the first to cross the threshold in the New Year. He or she usually bore gifts. Our front door was mainly glass and Dr Smith had had a little too much to drink. He fell through the glass door. My parents were furious especially my father who was a teetotaller. Dr Smith died at the young age of forty-seven.

The surgery had two consulting rooms, a waiting room and a room they called the dispensary. That room was where all the records were kept and was also reception. My father rarely kept written records. There was a door from reception into the private house. Patients used the downstairs lavatory in our house. Miss Gray was the receptionist in the early 1950s. Later receptionists Sylvia Ellerby and Joan Calvert are still very active at the time of writing. Joan Calvert became practice manager of the doctors working in the Henry Moore Clinic, and I was pleased to be asked to her retirement dinner. (That was the practice Dr Gilfillan started.) I met Mrs Ellerby in 2010 at the Methodist church in Altofts where I was giving a talk.

Miss Gray and my mother wore white coats. My father wore a three-piece suit for work, usually peppered with cigarette ash. The wearing of white coats by doctors continued until the 1970s.

The surgery was very small indeed. In the middle of an influenza epidemic, patients had to queue out into the street in the rain. One of those patients was a local alderman of the council. He complained that the surgery was too small and his views hit the local press. My parents won their case to keep the surgery as it was by obtaining the support of the Local Medical Committee. It certainly was far too small for 10,000 patients.

In 1957, there was the Asian Flu Epidemic. Both my parents were bedridden by the flu. Mrs McGrath, their housekeeper, saw the patients in the surgery, came up to the bedroom, and my parents would write out a prescription or absence from work certificate. I shudder to think what the General Medical Council would have to say about that.

House visits were a huge feature of general practice in the thirty years after the creation of the NHS. My parents would spend part of the evening updating a large ledger in which was kept lists of patients who required revisiting the next day. The phone would start ringing at about 8 a.m., and there would be scores of new visit requests to be undertaken as well as the revisits. There were two people living in different parts of the housing estate who also took messages and visit requests. This was because a large number of patients did not have telephones and the telephone boxes were often vandalised. The GP could park his or her car at the address of one visit and do a further six without driving. Visits were undertaken in all weathers and at all times. My father once walked over a mile to an evening visit request in the dense fog. The patient thanked him and told him that it would have been OK to leave it to the next day.

My parents' half day was on Thursday afternoon and this coincided with my half day when I was at school in Wakefield. If Dr Smith was not on holiday, they were free to do anything. We usually went out for lunch. In the summer we went to Monk Fryston Hall Hotel, which is in a beautiful setting with waterways crossed by ancient bridges. Often Lord and Lady Docker dined there. They were very ostentatious. Their Rolls Royce had stars embedded in the bodywork made of real gold. We sometimes went for lunch in Leeds at a restaurant called Jacomelli in Boar Lane. We often saw Herbert Sutcliffe, the famous Yorkshire-born MCC cricketer. After lunch, we might go to a cinema in Leeds. If Dr Smith was on holiday, my parents still closed the surgery but were on call. We might go to the Albion cinema in Castleford. On one occasion soon after the film had started, a message was projected on to the screen—'Phone call for Dr Sloan'. My father left and did a visit, returning to see the end of the film.

Of course my parents took their holidays at the same time, and this required employing a locum. Locums were quite expensive and sometimes not very good as doctors. One prescribed a blood pressure-lowering drug for all sorts of conditions unrelated to hypertension. Another had such poor vision that he had to be driven. The huge mounds of discarded rubble from the mining of coal were called muck stacks. The locum with poor vision thought these were beautiful mountains.

Airedale was a deprived area at that time and, despite significant improvements, still is. My mother took me around in her car shortly before Christmas delivering mince pies to poor families. This was in the evening and it was pitch dark. We arrived at one house, and I thought there was no one in because there were no lights on. My mother explained that this was Mr and Mrs Stevens and they were both blind. They later became my patients when I started work in Castleford.

In the 1950s and to a lesser extent as the decades went on, it was not unheard of for women to have six, seven, or eight children. I know of one father who did not realise his wife was pregnant for about the eighth time, asking her where she was going when she set off to the maternity home in labour. My mother undertook most of the obstetric work. There was a maternity home in Castleford and the weekly antenatal clinic in the surgery took all afternoon. The longest standing midwife was Edna Box. She developed a close relationship with my mother. After my father died, they went on holiday together as Edna was also widowed. Edna brought her very young son, Timothy, to the house when she was working with my mother in the antenatal clinic. My father would babysit in the house while the clinic took place in the surgery.

The relationship of GPs with consultants has radically changed in the last sixty years. Now GPs hardly meet consultants. The domiciliary home visit by a consultant was very popular from the inception of the NHS until the start of the 1990s. The GP phoned the consultant and asked him or her to visit one of their patients to give an opinion. This might be a case that the GP did not want to admit to hospital and who needed an expert opinion. I remember, as a child, consultants arriving at the house and having a cup of tea or even something stronger with my parents. The psychiatrist, Dr Fenton-Russell was a regular visitor. My mother or father would accompany the consultant to the house of the patient where an assessment was made and an opinion given. This took significant time. When I started working as a GP, joint visits did take place but these were replaced by the consultant visiting alone. My mother had a close professional relationship with a cardiologist, John Turner. Indeed, she was somewhat in awe of the status of consultants. I always felt I was a disappointment by becoming 'only' a GP. When my mother developed diabetes, Dr Turner dealt with this for her over the telephone. I also developed a very good professional relationship with him when I started as a GP in Castleford.

There was only one chemist (pharmacy) in Airedale up until about 1960. Mr Carter was the pharmacist and my parents were friends of the Carters. They would come to the house and played poker with my mother. My father did not play cards or gamble and often went to bed early. He used to come downstairs in his pyjamas to say goodnight to them. My mother also loved roulette. I have spent significant time, with my father, waiting outside casinos or in the car if my mother was on a winning streak in there. Her father was a very significant gambler. Forgive me if I digress a little here. My grandparents once went on a holiday from Berlin to Monte Carlo. My grandfather was having such a good run of wins that the family travelled back home at the end of the holiday leaving him at the casino. His favourite numbers were 8, 11, and 30 with sometimes 17. Only those familiar with roulette will understand that one can use two chips to bet on 8, 11, and 30 because 8 and 11 are adjacent on the layout. The numbers 8, 11, and 30 are next to one another on the wheel. These are the only numbers like that. When he had a huge win in Monte Carlo, he put a huge amount of money on 17. It won and he left the winnings on 17 and it won again.

General practice partnerships are like a marriage. Eventually my parents fell out with Dr Smith. They would not let him in the house to use the lavatory and he used a chemical lavatory in a room off the garage. I do not know what all this was about. Eventually, Dr Smith was persuaded to leave the partnership by my father retiring and allowing Dr Smith to take all the patients registered with my father (perhaps a few thousands). A great number of these patients came back to join my mother's list. Indeed, there were so many at first that she used a shopping basket in which she collected all the medical cards. She advertised for a new partner. At that time, in the early 1960s, it was very difficult to get a partner. My parents bought a house and the advert included the successful applicant living in that house rent and rates free. My father was so excited when an almost perfect application came in. However, this turned out to be fictitious and written by his brother Sam who was a GP in the nearby town of Wakefield. My mother took on Dr Suniel Minocha. He was married to Devika, an anaesthetist. My father continued to work with my mother for no income. His title was 'honorary unpaid assistant'.

My father's brother Samuel's appearance and behaviour was a contrast to my father's. He smartly dressed in a three-piece suit and wore a French beret when out on visits and the weather was inclement. In cold weather, he used a pair of gloves that could be heated up electrically by plugging them into the cigar lighter socket of his car. This was so his hands were always warm for examining patients. He started in general practice in Helperby, North Yorkshire, but fell out with his partner who was up to no good. Partnership problems have been relatively common right up to the present time.

From the age of six, I went to Queen Elizabeth Grammar School, Wakefield. I joined the cubs and then the boy scouts there. The scout meetings were weekly in the late afternoon going into early evening. After the scout meeting, I would stay at Uncle Sam's house in Wakefield. I loved staying there, and I once told my parents, 'I like Wakefield better than England'. (Geography was not a strong subject of mine.) Uncle Sam's wife, Agnes, is, along with their daughter, Angela, my only

Yorkshire relatives. Aunty Agnes was great fun and had a great laugh. Angela is slightly older than me and she went to the sister school of mine, Wakefield Girl's High School. When she was young, the families got together a lot. I had a crush on Angela at some point and looked up whether cousins could marry. Angela had left home to study medicine at Queens University, Belfast, by the time I started staying at the Wakefield house.

Sam was in partnership with three others based at the Warrengate Surgery in central Wakefield. A difference of opinion occurred and my uncle practised as a virtual single-handed GP from a small surgery attached to their house. My father was a chain-smoker. Uncle Sam smoked three cigarettes a day, one after each meal, which I thought very civilised. Gladys was their housekeeper, and there was a gong in the hall, which she used to summon people to meals. I loved having a go on the gong. Before breakfast, I had to clean my uncle's shoes. They thought this would do me good as back in Castleford as our housekeeper cleaned the shoes. The shoes I cleaned were black and were bought and used by Sam's father, my grandfather.

Breakfast was taken in the dining room at a rather large dining table and my uncle sat at the head of it. He opened his mail neatly with a letter opener. Some of the envelopes contained cheques, which were share dividends. My father opened his post while still in bed. He certainly did not use a letter opener but rather ripped the envelopes apart. GPs received lots of adverts from drug companies. He used to throw these away without opening them. He once threw away his quarterly pay cheque. My uncle was one of the very few doctors at that time who accumulated sufficient money such that he could retire at sixty instead of sixty-five. My father retired early at the age of sixty-three and my mother when she became sixty-five. After he retired, my father told us that his NHS pension paid for my mother's supertax. GPs were very well paid up until the mid-1960s.

Sometimes I would spend the afternoon of my school half day with Uncle Sam and Aunty Agnes. We would often go out to the countryside and have a picnic. This was sometimes in North Yorkshire or the Yorkshire Dales. One objective of the picnic was that the site should have no signs of human habitation. This was a moderate challenge in the late 1950s and early 1960s. It is a really tough challenge now.

After Angela qualified, she married John and had two children, Alison and Nick. They seemed settled in Northern Ireland. Soon after the Northern Irish troubles began there, the family emigrated to Brisbane, Australia. I was honoured to be asked to be Nick's godfather. He too became a doctor but gave up medicine to pursue a successful career as a novelist. My uncle and aunt had retired to Northern Ireland, and it must have been a shock for their only daughter and grandchildren to emigrate so far away. Eventually, after my uncle died, Agnes emigrated to Brisbane. She was then in her early eighties. She celebrated her ninetieth birthday there and thoroughly enjoyed her new life.

At one point in my early life, I wanted to be a Church of England vicar. This was in my early teens. After that, I never faltered in my desire to become a doctor and a GP in particular. There was never any pressure on me from my parents to pass examinations or pursue a medical career. I loved the way of life of the GP. My parents bought me a Hillman Imp car to take to London when I left home. I did not realise how upset a parent would be with an only child leaving home. They never showed any signs to me of upset.

CHAPTER 2

PRECLINICAL MEDICAL STUDENT

Let me explain what a preclinical medical student is. At the time I became a medical student in 1962, there were two stages to go through before qualifying as a doctor. The second stage was called 'clinical', and the learning was largely with patients on the wards of a teaching hospital. The first eighteen months of study was called 'preclinical', and we were taught anatomy, physiology, biochemistry, and pharmacology by means of lectures and practical sessions. We very rarely saw any patients during that time.

Three friends (Colin Teasdale, Kevin Pavey, and myself) were in the sixth form of Queen Elizabeth Grammar School, Wakefield, West Yorkshire, and we decided that we wanted to go to London to study medicine. We would have had to stay on for a third year in the sixth form to go to Oxford or Cambridge universities. The headmaster wanted us to do that. (I found out later that the pay of the headmaster was determined by the number of students he had in the sixth form). We decided to apply to the London Hospital Medical College in Whitechapel—the East End of London. For me, one reason for that choice was that the medical school was situated near the docks in the East End of London and, the other, it had a large number of hospital beds. Being near the docks ensured some rare diseases brought in by immigrants. These included tropical diseases. There were also significant cases of asbestosis (there was an asbestos factory in the East End). Because of the large number of beds, there were plenty of patients for each student to study.

The interviews at the London for Colin and me were on the same day, and we travelled down to London together. Colin's interview was timed to be the one before mine. We smartened ourselves up in the gentlemen's lavatory at Kings Cross railway station. It was a rainy day, and when we emerged from the station, a lorry drove past and splashed mud and water up on one of my trouser legs. You will see below why I have always maintained that Colin pushed me so that I would be splattered with mud for the interview and so give him an advantage. Of course he did not push me and the splashing was an accident.

We were interviewed by Dr John Ellis, later to become dean, and Mr Jack Crawford, the medical sub-dean. Dr Ellis was a physician and Mr Crawford a neurosurgeon. Colin was called in first. One of them asked him, 'Who you think is the better student, you or Richard Sloan?' He answered that he thought it was himself. I was then called in and asked the same question. I answered that I thought it was Colin. Colin was offered a place and I was not. He definitely pushed me! My other friend from school, Kevin Pavey, also got a place at the London.

My second choice was University College, London, and its hospital. I was interviewed by Dr Datta, a biochemist. After several questions, he was staring at my application form and exclaimed, 'What the hell's this? Mr Bagley! He taught me on the Isle of Wight.' Mr Bagley was the headmaster of my school. I was accepted as a student. On each of the application forms to the various medical schools, I had indicated that I would be willing to start in either 1962 or 1963. If I started in September 1962, I would only have been seventeen years of age, my birthday being in November. It was generally accepted that one had to be 18 to go to university. Dr Datta was happy with me starting sooner rather than later.

I also applied to Guy's Hospital and on the application form was a question, 'What position do you play in rugby union?' I absolutely hated rugby but answered 'fullback'. I was never even asked for an interview. Presumably, a lot of fullbacks applied that year.

Being accepted as a medical student today is so very different from what it was like in 1962. Now, one has to apply using the Universities and Colleges Admissions Service (UCAS). There is only a very small area on the application form for a personal statement where one can write about hobbies and so on. Advice on how to complete the form is given in detail on the UCAS Web site. The A-level requirements now are either three A grades or two As and one B. It is rare that a medical school will accept one A and two Bs. The Leeds Widening Access to Medical School Scheme has a Web site called 'So you want to be a doctor', which gives detailed advice on how to perform best at an interview. One should read up on medical issues and ethics, learn about the NHS, and be familiar with the medical news. There is guidance on body language, how to enter and leave the room, and what to wear (boys should wear black socks!).

What a contrast with 1962! We applied to medical school via the Universities Central Council on Admissions (UCCA), which had been established in 1961. One listed one's preferred medical school. I wanted to go to a London medical school. The A level requirements were three passes, preferably in biology, physics, and chemistry. My school taught us how to prepare for the interview. The headmaster undertook mock interviews with us three who wanted to go to London and first had us in his room to brief us. He told me that when he asks me the question 'Why do you want to become a doctor?', I should *not* answer 'because both my parents are doctors'. He sent us out. When he called me in, the first question he asked me was 'Why do you want to become a doctor?' I answered, 'Because both my parents are doctors and I like their way of life'. It was the truth, but he was not at all pleased.

The school gave us a huge reading list consisting mainly of works of fiction that we were to read in the summer holidays. I enjoyed reading these novels, and I knew that what I had read might come up in my interview. Sports and hobbies were also important. All applicants to medical schools in the UK were interviewed and the interview was paramount.

Over the years, there has been a trend away from three ordinary passes in A levels to three very high grades being required to enter medical school. I feel this is a retrogressive step. My experience in postgraduate general practice education backs this up. Do we want doctors who can cram and are good at exams or do we want rounded cultured doctors taking the holistic approach? Does one have to be so bright to become a doctor? I believe not. For A levels, I obtained grade As in Physics and Biology and obtained a B in Chemistry. (My chemistry master told me off for performing so poorly.) I got a D in General Studies. I failed S-level biology by writing on the wrong subject for one question. Superficially, it looks as though I was a 'crammer'. However, I had superb teaching at Queen Elizabeth Grammar School, Wakefield. In mock A levels, I might get 70 per cent on a paper and some of my fellow students 95 per cent. All of us got A grades. This demonstrates a flaw in the marking system. I am convinced that my contemporaries at medical school have had more fulfilled careers and a broader medical and general education than the doctors qualifying in later years.

The closest anyone got to a student loan in those days was contracting with one section of the armed forces to work for it for a number of years after qualification in exchange for a monthly allowance as an undergraduate. This monthly allowance was much higher than the student grant. One of my friends, John McCardy did this, but bought himself out of the army later to become a GP in Ireland. He certainly had more money than us when we were students. There was a means tested grant awarded to all students in the UK. I had the minimum termly grant of £50 as my parents earned well as GPs. My parents made this grant up to the approximately £110 a term, which was the amount of full grant each student should have. A term was roughly ten weeks, and we could live in London for about £10 a week. The rent on one flat in which I lived was £2.50 per week and a loaf of bread and a pint of beer cost about 5p each. One of my student friends bought a second hand van for £10. The amount £110 then is worth roughly £1,600 in today's money. In 2010, student debt was predicted to be about £25,000 and the rise in tuition fees proposed in 2011 could make this even more, despite repayments being lessened. I would not like to have had a huge loan to pay off at the start of my career, even if the interest rates and repayment levels were low. In 2010, there were approximately 480,000 students admitted to universities in the UK. It would cost the taxpayer 4.32 billion pounds to pay £9,000 tuition fees for each one for a year. The defence budget for 2011 is approximately 40 billion pounds. I think you can guess my train of thought on this subject.

The preclinical teaching at University College London (UCL) was separate from University College Hospital, which was across the road (Gower Street). The preclinical departments were part of the university. There were about 120 students in our intake. We could attend any lectures that were taking place in the university, and we mixed with students from other departments. Indeed, John Popper, the cousin of my good friend George Goodenough back home, started at UCL at the same time as me. John was studying Geography. It appeared to me that he had to attend about three lectures each week and then rest of the week was free. This was in contrast to preclinical medical students who had a packed programme of learning. I was pleased to be part of a proper university rather than doing this part of my studying at a medical college such as the London Hospital Medical College. There were separate departments of Anatomy, Physiology, Biochemistry, and Pharmacology at the London, but I think the preclinical students there felt very much part of the hospital. There were dental and medical students as well as student nurses at the London. Kings College was the only other place in London, where medical students started in a university.

UCL held evening debates, and I went to one where David Frost was one of the debaters. There were also debates held in the University of London Union (ULU) building that was just round the corner. There was a great book shop nearby with an excellent range of medical text books. I joined the shooting club, and there was a firing range on site. University College was left wing. I remember going to a General Election Hustings, and there was a crowd from UCL. Quintin Hogg (later Lord Hailsham) was speaking. When he started to speak and said, 'We in the conservative party do not think . . .', he was interrupted by a chant, 'we do not think, we do not think'. It was one of the few times I saw him flustered. There were some seriously famous academics at UCL at that time. It was a privilege for us to have two of these as our teachers (J. Z. Young and Andrew Huxley).

A large part of the anatomy curriculum was dissecting a human body. On the first day we were shown around the dissection room, and some of the 120 students of that year's intake were very nervous about seeing a dead body. I did not feel too badly about it. There was a strong smell of formaldehyde. (I have a photograph of my mother in her dissecting room in Berlin and she is smoking a pipe). Six students were allocated to a body, and we were divided up alphabetically. The surnames of the students on our dissection table all began with 'S'—Sloan, Smith, Smeeton, Singleton-Turner, and so on. Grahame Smith and Jim Smeeton became two of my closest friends. The friendships that started around the dissection table were the best thing that dead body did for me.

The first lecture was by professor of anatomy, John Zacchary Young (known as JZ), and to this day I remember what he said to us in that lecture.

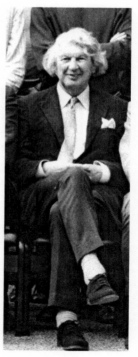

The lecture was partly about a physiological topic, which was a bit of a shock at the time as he was a professor of anatomy. He told us about a nineteenth-century physiologist, Paul Bernard, who wrote, 'La fixité du milieu intérieur est la condition d'une vie libre et indépendante'. (The constancy of the internal environment is the condition for a free and independent life.) This is homeostasis, which is the mechanism a body maintains a stable interior independent of the changes in the external environment. For example, the deep body temperature is generally maintained around 37°C in both hot and cold climates. In that lecture, he also told us about the significance of the invention of the printing press on science.

JZ Young

JZ did not have a medical degree but was seriously eminent, having delivered the second BBC Reith lecture. He was the vice president of the Royal Society.

At first I found the thought of having to learn so much a daunting prospect. I found the long words very difficult. For example, eosinophilic, polymorphic, leucocyte (a cell) and levator labii alaeqi nasi (a muscle). At the same time, there were some pretty articulate students with posh accents and some with double-barrelled surnames. I thought they all must be much brighter than me. I came to the conclusion that I was probably in the bottom 50 per cent and would have to work really hard to get through. I actually lost some weight with the anxiety of all this.

The preclinical study of anatomy was divided between lectures, dissection, and some practical sessions dealing with histology slides and embryology.

We each had to buy half a skeleton and a whole skull. I took the purchase back to our flat in a carrier bag on the underground and was careful not to have an accident and spill the bones on to the carriage floor. Using the bible of human anatomy, Gray's Anatomy, and with dissection sessions, we learnt about every single muscle, bone, artery, vein, nerve, organ, and more of the body. Each term we dissected a different part of the body. For example, we dissected the head and neck one term and the abdomen another. Each week we would be tested by a doctor called an anatomy demonstrator. I think these doctors were lecturers in anatomy. There is a complicated junction of nerves in the armpit called the brachial plexus and between us, by mistake, we managed to completely destroy it. We were in a panic because we thought we would get into trouble when the demonstrator came around. Grahame Smith found a tendon, which we were going to throw away and made a brilliant brachial plexus out of it and placed it in the armpit. We fooled the demonstrator completely. Or did we?

Like the first lecture by JZ, some of the other lecturers in anatomy were very broad in their approach because of the interesting research they were undertaking. I remember one who was an expert on moles who told us how they had vestigial eyes covered with skin and hairs. They were blind. He explained how they found their way around using their whiskers.

Histology was difficult. (Actually, everything was difficult for me.) We were taught about how tissues were sliced very thinly and stained. When I first looked down a microscope, I could not see anything apart from my eyelashes. We had to train our eyes to look in a particular way. Eventually, it all became clear. I was entering the world of the very small. We learnt how to recognise arteries, veins, and nerves in cross section on the slides as well as differentiating organs such as liver and kidney. The preclinical course was teaching us about the body in its normal state. The thoughts of later having to recognise down the microscope diseased tissue such as cancer, infection, and so on in slides with areas of normal cells brought me out in a sweat. There were some great text books of histology with pictures that were a tremendous help. We had lectures on histology as well.

Electron microscopy was newish in those days, and a lot of research using this type of microscope was going on in the anatomy department. Light microscopes can magnify about 200 times but electron microscopes 2,000,000 times or so. There was a Ph.D. student who was studying the electron microscopy of the rudimentary auditory apparatus (ear) of glow worms. The colour pictures produced by electron microscopes are particularly beautiful. In 2008, I visited the department of anatomy, and there were framed photographs of electron microscope slides on the walls of the stairway. They were in colour and fabulous to look at.

We also had anatomy tutorials. There were about eight students in each tutorial group. With a good teacher, tutorials were a great opportunity to learn not only from the tutor but also from one another.

Physiology is the study of how the normal body works. Of course, one cannot learn physiology without a knowledge of anatomy. Physiology teaching was by lectures, which sometimes included practical demonstrations by the lecturers, tutorials, and practical classes. The head of department was Prof. Andrew Huxley, who was an expert on the physiology of how nerves conduct electricity. He continued to undertake research and teach until his death in May 2012 at the age of 94.

We found his lectures somewhat boring and used to count how many times he said 'erm'. For one term, he was our physiology tutor. There were about eight of us in that tutorial group. After a practical class, we had to write up the experiment in a book, which we handed in to our tutor to be marked. Professor Huxley had the most amazing brain and intellect, and I was a bit frightened of him. He knew the logarithm tables by heart and learnt to speak Russian in a few weeks in order to go on a lecture tour. He marked our practical books and gave us feedback. When the announcement was made that Professor Huxley had won the Nobel Prize for medicine in 1963 for discovering how nerves worked, he became an immediate star. After that, his lectures were packed with students from every department of University College. I remember one such lecture when he inserted an electrode into a muscle of his forearm and showed the electrical activity going on when he contracted it.

The experiments we did in the practical sessions included measuring our urine output after drinking an amount of water with and without an injection of antidiuretic hormone. We had to continue measuring this in the evening when we had returned to our flat. We also did experiments on pithed frogs. A pithed frog has had its spinal cord cut in the neck so it is insensible. I hated this. Another experiment was studying the heartbeat of a tortoise that had been dissected such that a hook could be inserted into the heart muscle and then recordings made of its movement by means of a cord from the hook to a smoked drum. Tortoise hearts beat very slowly, and we looked at the effects of some drugs such as adrenalin on the heart rate. I found physiology very interesting as by understanding how the body works normally, one should be able to work out what is happening when it goes wrong due to a disease.

Biochemistry was another subject, and I actually learnt most of a textbook of biochemistry by heart. When it came to the exams, I could even remember the page numbers. One of the textbooks mentioned my mother's uncle, Ernst Friedman, who left Germany to become a professor of biochemistry at Cambridge University. One of the most important biochemical processes we had to learn was the Krebs cycle. This was a series of chemical reactions that took place that enabled oxygen to be used by cells. It was a very complicated cycle of reactions and difficult to learn. One of my friends, Mike Dawson, when asked to describe the Krebs cycle in the biochemistry examination at the London Hospital Medical College, wrote 'The Krebs cycle is far too difficult to commit to memory and I haven't'. He failed and was thrown out but eventually was allowed to continue his studies. He became a successful orthopaedic surgeon in the USA. At the end of the eighteen-month preclinical period, there was a five-hour biochemistry practical examination. I finished this after two hours and walked out. I then got into a panic that I had missed something, but I hadn't. I passed.

The fourth subject we were taught in the first eighteen months at medical school was pharmacology. This was the only subject for one was allowed to fail and continue with one's clinical studies. The examination could be retaken during the early part of clinical studies. The head of the department was Prof. Heinz Otto Schild. He had a heavy Austrian accent. We used to mock him saying things like 'ven I vas doing research in Germany experimenting on huma ... I mean rabbits'. I remember a notice advertising an evening dance that had on it 'Come and knock the 'ell out of Schild' (pronounced shilt). He was a very good teacher, and I did not realise how eminent he was until I read his obituary in the *British Medical Journal* published in 1984. He was a doctor of medicine, a doctor of philosophy, a doctor of science, and a Fellow of the Royal Society. Like my mother, he had to leave Germany, where he was working, because of the Nazi threat. He was an expert on histamine and drug antagonists. Another excellent teacher was Prof. D. R. Laurence. He wrote a book called *Clinical Pharmacology*, which is a salient work. Pharmacology was of supreme importance to us as I am sure one can help patients better if one understood the basics of drug actions rather than learning lists of indications, interactions, and side effects.

We had practical pharmacology teaching and these classes usually lasted all afternoon. We worked in pairs and my partner was Grahame Smith. One experiment involved each of us swallowing a tablet, letting it act, and then measuring things such as doing a maths exercise or a memory test. One of us had been given an amphetamine (speed) tablet and the other a barbiturate (a sedative). We were not told what the drugs were. Grahame got quite irritated with me and wanted to rush on. I was being so slow and couldn't be bothered doing anything. The measurements were such that we could prove that one of us had been given a sedative and the other a stimulant. The objective of that teaching was to make us appreciate blind experimentation and to record observations in a formal way. It was also fun. Grahame has kept the book where he recoded all the results. I am not sure that those experiments with students would get through an ethical committee today.

Another pharmacology practical was definitely unethical. My fellow medical student and flatmate Steve Haggie was given the drug hexamethonium. It was used to lower blood pressure. On researching this drug on the Internet, I came across a discussion group and one person wrote 'side effects is too mild a term for hexamethonium'. The drug blocks all automatic nerves like those that control blood pressure, the bowels, and so on. For example, after taking hexamethonium, if one is lying down and an arm is raised up, the blood drains out and the arm goes white. Steve ended up with virtually no blood pressure and feeling faint when he stood up. He had to be virtually carried home on the underground train and recovered later in the evening.

The examination we had to pass at the end of the eighteen months of preclinical study was called second MB (Bachelor of Medicine). The third MB was the final examination. There was an examination called first MB, and this was for students who had not attained the requisite A levels at school—physics, chemistry, and biology. Some medical schools, such as St Mary's Hospital Medical School, Paddington, took in students for a year to study one or more of these subjects. I was absolutely petrified of the examination for second MB. We knew that out of our year, about twenty would fail. Last thing at night, my flatmates and I used to try and think of twenty people who were more likely to fail than us. Grahame sometimes could only get to nineteen, and in order to get to sleep, he added himself as the twentieth. I therefore worked very hard for this examination.

The results were to be posted up on a notice board one late afternoon. My flatmates and I decided to go to the cinema in the early afternoon to take our minds off things. The film was the *Ipcress File* with Michael Caine. After the film, we went back to the university to get our results. It was horrible looking at the lists of names that had passed biochemistry, anatomy, physiology, and pharmacology. If your name was missing, you had failed. It was difficult to see the lists because of the crowding around the notice board. I passed all four subjects and was thrilled. We were so upset that one of our flatmates, Colin Parker, had failed some of the subjects. He would have to spend another term studying and retake. Those who came in the top 20 per cent could apply to spend an extra eighteen months studying to achieve a B.Sc. in one of the four preclinical subjects. To my surprise, I was one of these and applied to do a B.Sc. in anatomy and was accepted. Why did I choose anatomy? Part of the course involves spending six weeks of the summer holiday with J. Z. Young in the Stazione Zoologica in Naples, Italy, helping him with his research. I was very fortunate that my parents were willing to continue funding me for this extra study. Indeed, I would not have been able to achieve most of the academic side of my career without the most generous support from my parents and after my father died, my mother.

So far in this chapter, I have concentrated on describing the academic journey to passing the second MB, but as everyone who has been to university knows, there is also life to learn about. London was a fantastic place to be in the 1960s, and despite working hard at my studies, I had a mostly thoroughly enjoyable time.

I really did not appreciate until later in life what a heart-wrenching experience it must have been for my parents, particularly my mother, for me to leave home to go to London. They bought me a Hillman Imp car, which was very generous. Colin Teasdale and I had arranged to go into digs together in North London. At one point, we suspected the landlady was nosing about our things. I fixed cotton threads across drawers to see if this was so. It was. Colin complained to her about something, and from that point onwards, she served him a smaller plate of food for his evening meal compared with mine. Colin was a religious person and a member of the Plymouth Brethren sect. He regularly read the Bible to himself. I was a member of the British Humanist Society. I have always said that Colin remained religious until he saw the light. The light came in the form of life at the London Hospital Medical College and that included life in the Good Samaritan public house. I used to drive from the digs to University College every day. I have never particularly enjoyed going on the underground train. In November, the smog arrived in most of the UK's big cities and in particular London. One night I could not see to drive home and stayed with friends of my parents in Roehampton. I did not phone Mrs Fisher, and she was rightly angry with me. One evening, we saw her sneaking out wearing a uniform. She was in the Salvation Army. We could only stand one term of these digs, and after that Colin and I went our separate ways and lived in rented flats. I think Colin complained about those first digs to the University of London.

I was allowed to drink legally in a pub only after my eighteenth birthday on 26 November. I took no notice of that. I remember one of my school friends telling me he had celebrated his eighteenth birthday in a Yorkshire Dales pub with a gang of friends all of whom were under eighteen. I started smoking cigarettes in that term. Up until then, I had occasionally stolen my father's cigarette tab ends and smoked the tobacco in a pipe. I became rapidly addicted and smoked at least twenty cigarettes a day until I stopped smoking at the age of about forty. When I went home for a weekend in the middle of that term, my father immediately offered me a cigarette as soon as I sat down with him. He knew his son. A lot of the students smoked and most enjoyed drinking a lot of alcohol. Like most students, I took my dirty washing home mid-term. Once I posted my dirty washing to my mother! I telephoned my parents regularly and reversed the charges.

After the digs, I moved into a one-room flat with Jim Smeeton. The flat was just off Baker Street. The bathroom was shared with another flat. On the first evening there, we were settling down to read, and I asked Jim what his book was. It was the Bible. I couldn't believe I was with another deeply religious person. Then he got his knitting out! Jim became a great friend. He came from Lancing, and I met his mother on several occasions, his father having passed away. Jim died not so long ago, and while clearing out his things, his widow, Liz, found a premium bond in my name and sent it to me. I was a bit broken at one time and sold half the premium bond to Jim. Half a premium bond was worth 50p. I wrote to Liz to tell her that if it wins, I will share the winnings with her. We only spent one term there and then a gang of four of us looked for a more spacious flat.

In the first summer holidays, a group of us rented a house on the island of St Mary in the Scilly Isles. It was idyllic and we went on boat trips to the other islands. We went to a James Bond film in an ancient cinema, and the entrance ticket was one shilling and threepence. The seas could be very rough and travelling between islands exciting. We repeated this holiday after we had taken the second MB examination. The boat crossing from the mainland was very rough indeed. I prided myself as a good sailor, and when the others were feeling queasy, I went below to the bar to have a drink. I was the only one there, and before the barman had finished pouring my beer, he had to rush off and be sick himself. Steve Haggie is a great birdwatcher, and to his annoyance, I often remind him of an event that happened on that holiday in the Scilly Isles to this day. He heard a tweeting sound around a corner and diagnosed it as a lesser-spotted-something bird. When we turned the corner, we discovered the noise coming from two twigs rubbing against one another.

The four in the new flat were Jim Smeeton, Grahame Smith, Steve Haggie, and myself. We found a place in Powis Terrace in Notting Hill Gate. At that time, Peter Rachman was a landlord made famous by exploiting his tenants, which were mainly in Notting Hill. I don't think he was our landlord, but one Sunday our street was splashed all over the front page of a tabloid newspaper with a story of some sex scandal going on in one of Rachman's properties in our street. His exploitation method became known as 'Rachmanism'. The flat had mice and each of us bought a mousetrap and had a competition as to who caught the most. One night a mouse was trapped while shutting the bedroom door. In the end, we got the rat man in to sort this out. The bedroom had four single beds, and one night one of the others tied some cotton to the corner of my pillow. As I was nodding off, someone tugged on the cotton. Of course I thought it was a mouse and jumped out of my skin. The others maintained I talked in my sleep and tried to record me. We were studying for the second MB and Grahame developed a habit just before we turned the bedroom light out of telling us his 'thought for the night'. Examples of these were adrenalin, the sciatic nerve, the bones of the ear, engine oil, and so on.

I had the Hillman Imp and Grahame bought himself an old van. At that point, neither Jim nor Steve had a car. We had great fun with Grahame's van. We offered to pay him £10 to push the thing over the white cliffs of Dover. He loved that van dearly. There was a particular bend somewhere in Paddington that Grahame took at a very fast speed such that it was very frightening to be a passenger. We called it 'the bend'. We often went with Grahame for a drive solely to experience 'the bend'. The engine of the van had to be started using a starting handle inserted at the front of the vehicle. One evening we decided to go for a ride in the van wearing our pyjamas. We knew that if Grahame stalled the engine, one of us would have to get out and start it up with the handle. It did not stall, but when we got back to the flat, there was not a single parking space in our street and we had to park in the next one and run home in our pyjamas. This was worse than having to start the engine with a handle. We often went on long trips in the van at the weekends taking girlfriends with us.

One evening I lent Jim my Hillman Imp to take his girlfriend Claire to Paddington station to catch a train to Reading, where she was studying maths. The next morning my car was missing, and I reported the theft to the police. We did not hear anything, and after about five days, Steve pointed out that there was a Hillman Imp of the same colour as mine part in our street and that this car had not moved for five days. I tried my car keys and they fitted both the door and ignition of that car. What had happened was that Jim had driven home from Paddington station in a different Hillman Imp the same colour as mine. Of course someone had reported their Hillman Imp stolen from Paddington station. It was all sorted out in the end. I once drove the Hillman Imp from Castleford to Harpenden (163 miles) in two hours flat with no one on the A1 overtaking me.

There was a gang of us who did things together like going to parties and dances. Geof Mair, Steve Haggie, Grahame Smith, Gill English, Abdul Palliwalla, Sheila Hall, Jenny Voke, Colin Parker, Diana Norkett, and Jim Smeeton were the main members of the group.

We went out for meals and had a favourite Indian restaurant. There was one restaurant in Leicester Square called the Guinea and Piggy, where for 21 shillings (a guinea) one could eat as much as one wanted. We starved ourselves one weekend and then stuffed our faces. We went to classical music concerts in the Albert Hall and Festival Hall. There were university clubs. I joined a shooting club—target shooting. Grahame was in the rowing club. Most of us had girl/boyfriends at this stage.

Steve went out with Gill and they eventually got married and they now live in Rotherham. Steve became a consultant surgeon and Gill a family planning clinician. Steve never had a single private patient, which is unique.

I went out with Diana Norkett for a while. She was and is a lovely person. She became a GP. We split up when I met my now wife Kath, who was a student at Kings College. Jim went out with Claire, a maths student at Reading University. She was seriously clever. In her final examination, there were a lot of questions and the instructions were 'Answer as many as you can'. She answered enough to be awarded a first-class degree and had enough extra marks that could have obtained an upper second as well. She went on to do a Ph.D. Jim became a GP.

Grahame, Colin, and Geof became GPs. Abdul went down the path of consultant paediatrician. He encountered serious racism. One consultant would talk to him only through a third person. He eventually became a GP. Jenny became a consultant haematologist. Sheila also became a consultant.

I spent quite a few days and evenings with close friends of my parents, Gerda (Beba) and Henry Tintner. They were GPs working in Roehampton. They were very kind to me feeding me and letting me take out their au pair girl to concerts.

My parents came to London regularly and treated my flatmates to meals out. They were very generous to me financially, buying me cars and giving me money. After the Hillman Imp, I had a sports car, a Triumph Spitfire. I was a very fortunate student indeed. Steve, Gill, and Grahame and his wife Caroline live near us now and remain close friends.

Kath was in the same hall of residence as a close friend of mine, Rosslynne Wheeldon, who was from Airedale, Castleford. Rosslynne introduced me to Kath. The hall of residence was called Nutford House. It was a female-only hall and there was a time that residents had to be back no later than 11 p.m. A lot of climbing in through windows went on.

I had a wonderful time in the first eighteen months in London despite the anxiety of studying and exams. After the exams, we had a great summer holiday.

After the summer holidays, six of us moved into a flat in Russell Road, near Olympia and off Kensington High Street. Colin Teasdale and Colin Parker joined the four of us who were in Powis Terrace.

CHAPTER 3

AN ANATOMY DEGREE

After the second MB examination, the next learning stage for most of the intake was to spend three years in University College Hospital as a clinical student learning about diseases, consulting with and examining patients, and learning how to prescribe. If one had done well in the second MB examination, one might be offered the opportunity to spend an extra eighteen months of study towards a B.Sc. (Special). Another exam! Between twenty and thirty students out of the 120 were offered a place on such a course. There was a choice of discipline and I chose anatomy rather than biochemistry, physiology, or pharmacology. My friend and flatmate Colin also chose to do an anatomy degree at the London Hospital Medical College. The disadvantage of studying for this extra time was that most of my friends would become doctors eighteen months before I would. One of the reasons I chose anatomy was that the course was run by J. Z. Young and involved a six-week trip to Naples, Italy, to undertake research with him and his team.

J. Z. Young (JZ) was a very famous scientist and prolific writer. He was appointed professor of anatomy at University College in the year of my birth, 1945. I would like to describe him and his work before outlining what we did on the course. The B.Sc. was a JZ degree.

In 1960 he published a book based on the Reith lectures he gave in 1950.[2] My favourite quote from that book is 'Whether we like it or not, we can be sure that societies that use to the full the new techniques of communication, by better language and by better machines, will eventually replace those that do not'. I think that could mean, for the evolution of man, there will be survival of the best communicators rather than survival of those with the most physical strength.

J.Z.Young wrote a chapter in 1975 in 'The Neurosciences: Paths of Discovery'. I particularly like one passage that discusses how scientists work.

> 'I did the dissection, Eccles the recording, whilst Granit sat on a deck chair. We were not quite sure of his function. Perhaps he was deciding what logical methods we were to use, though I doubt whether scientists really proceed in the way that philosophers of science seem to suppose. It is a banal truism that all scientific workers operate with some hypotheses, but this alone does not adequately describe the motivation or process of their activities. Eccles, Granit and I were certainly not doing the work on earthworms to try and disprove the hypothesis that nerve fibres conduct. We were groping our way, trying to find new material for study. Disparagers can say that this is not science, but we three seem to have been moderately successful scientists.'

This counters all the politically and scientific correctness that researchers are expected to embrace today.

JZ's appearance was unconventional. He had a mass of long somewhat unkempt hair that was parted on the right, the same as mine. In the UK, men's partings are usually on the left. Partings in Western Europe are generally on the right. He had a deformed upper incisor tooth. When he was working in the laboratory in Naples, he often wore a black laboratory coat rather than the conventional white one.

---

2   J. Z. Young. 1960. *Doubt and Certainty in Science: A Biologist's Reflection on the Brain*. Oxford University Press.

JZ was one of the three great 'medical' heroes who have greatly influenced my thoughts and approach to science and doctoring. (The other two were Bill Keatinge and Jamie Bahrami.) The thing that struck me as I got to know him better was that he treated his students as equals, despite his great eminence. An obituary was written by Anthony Tucker for the *Guardian* newspaper on Monday, 14 July 1997. Below are some extracts from that obituary.

'. . . JZ Young, who has died aged 90, was one of the most influential biologists of the 20th century. His work in the 1920s on the nature of nervous systems, signal transmission and nerve fibre structure provided a platform which led, a quarter of a century later, to a Nobel prize for Sir Andrew Huxley and Sir Alan Hodgkin for their work on nerve signals.

. . . Working with P B Medawar, Young developed a method of rejoining small peripheral nerves by means 'glue' of plasma, a method eventually modified and exploited in surgery.

. . . After the war, however, Young turned to investigating the central nervous system and the functions of the brain. Young showed that an octopus can be trained to respond in specific ways to different visual stimuli. He then went on to show where in the cephalopod this trained memory is stored.

. . . Young's a speculative books on brain function and behaviour reveal the huge scale and the inherent humility of his scientific thinking.

. . . His Gifford lectures embraced physiology, coding and communication, evolution and what, at that time, was the cutting edge of molecular genetics. They also range fearlessly into vast and only partly chartered areas like language, love, belief, dreaming, pleasure and play.

...Young might be thought of as the last great philosophical descendant of Charles Darwin.

... He became the 1928-29 Oxford scholar at the Naples Zoological Station, then one of the world leaders in marine biology. It was there, studying the autonomous nervous system of fish, that Young investigated the tube like structures which serve the muscles driving the squid's jet propulsion system. Although these 'tubes' had been observed 20 years earlier, Young showed that they are giant nerve fibers, up to 1000 times the diameter of normal nerves. The discovery of these large nerve fibres in squid and cuttlefish opened the way for direct laboratory investigation of nerve structure and function.

... His energy and intellectual grasp remained prodigious and, at that time of this death (aged 90), he was working with Marion Nixon on an entirely new book on the cephalopods.'

What did the anatomy course embrace? The areas covered were anthropology, embryology, and histology. We were encouraged to question everything.

JZ employed the Oxford tutorial system. A subject was set or a question posed and the student wrote an essay. The essay was handed in and marked by a tutor. There was then a one-to-one tutorial lasting about an hour and the essay was discussed. We changed tutors at the beginning of each term. I felt daunted when JZ was my tutor. However, as I have already mentioned, one of his great strengths was that he treated his students most civilly and there was mutual respect. This was one of the main attributes I took away from that course, and I hope I dealt with my patients and employees in a similar fashion. I will give an example of the sort of tasks that were set for the tutorials. I was given two scientific papers to read and critically appraise. One was written by Solly Zuckerman and the other by Jacob Bronowski. Each was about a tooth of an animal that was an evolutionary precursor of man namely *Australopithecus*. One of the papers argued that the tooth was ape like and the other more humanoid. This was all part of the anthropology course.

For some of the learning, we joined with anatomy students from the rest of the University of London who were studying for this degree. I mentioned earlier that Colin Teasdale, my flatmate and friend, was also doing this course at the London Hospital. There were about thirty anatomy students from the other medical schools in London. There were three at the London Hospital Medical College. Because I knew Colin so well, I got to know the other two very well and often studied with them.

One was Robin Harrod, a fellow Yorkshireman from Scarborough, and the other Adrian Bomford, who was brought up in Aden. Robin's father was an optician. Robin was seriously bright. Indeed he came top in the University of London in the B.Sc. exam. Colin was also very clever. I think they were simply swats with very good memories but that comment reflects some envy of their significant intellects. Robin hated missing anything to do with learning. On one occasion, we made a fictitious reading list, which included some obscure paper in an obscure journal that was housed in a library in Outer London. The object of this was to see whether Robin would rush off to find that paper. He did not fall for this. Adrian's father was a doctor and his uncle, a consultant physician at the London. Adrian and I went off at tangents and read all sorts of possibly irrelevant papers and books. I read articles about yawning and consciousness. Adrian spent a long time reading Marshal's physiology of reproduction, which described in graphic detail how such animals as giraffes and elephants copulated. Adrian and I got lower seconds for our degrees. However, this was a B.Sc. (Special), and we obtained high marks in the second MB to start with.

Most of us found the subject of anthropology the most interesting. JZ was the driver of this part of the degree. We had a tutor, John Napier, who spent a week surviving only using Stone Age tools. He lost weight with this experiment. He would arrive for his teaching sessions with a cardboard box full of ashtrays for us to use if we smoked. How things have changed over the years! We studied evolution, looked at models of skulls, and learnt about *Australopithecus, Pithecanthropus, Homo erectus,* java man, and tools. The Olduvai Gorge in East Africa was the major site of these skeletal remains that determined the story of evolution.

For part of our final examination, we were given a skull to identify. It turned out to be the skull of Piltdown man. This skull was 'discovered' in 1912 and was regarded as a missing link in the evolution of man. It was revealed as a hoax in 1953. What a rotten thing to put in an exam or was it?

We also studied histology and embryology. In histology, we learnt about the various stains used to highlight cell membranes and nuclei of cells, and so on. In embryology, we learnt how a human developed after fertilisation of the egg. We looked at the development of other animals, fish and birds—comparative embryology and the relation of embryology to evolution.

I have written in the first chapter about my German and Jewish background. I cannot remember the names of all twelve of us who studied anatomy at University College. There was Robert Tresman, Bob Reichenbach, and David Bromham. David became a gynaecologist in Leeds but tragically died at a young age a number of years ago. I have lost touch with all of them but remain close friends with the two who studied the B.Sc. at the London Hospital, namely, my school friend Colin Teasdale and my future medical partner, Robin Harrod.

The most memorable and important feature of the course was that six of the group went to Naples, Italy, for the first half of the summer holidays, to work with JZ on research on octopuses and squid. The remaining six students went for the second half of the holiday and I was in that group. There was a Ph.D. student and a very attractive zoology student called Lucy. We each fell a bit in love with her. There were also several scientists working with JZ coming from all parts of the world. I remember one of them telling JZ to f*   *   * off because he had the habit of coming up behind you as you were working and looking over your shoulder. All this research was paid for by a grant from the Office of Aerospace Research of the United States Air force and the Nuffield Foundation. The research took place in the Stazione Zoologica, which was on the seafront. It is a beautiful building housing the oldest aquarium in Europe.

In the main laboratory, there were tanks, with circulating sea water, each containing an octopus with the lid secured with bricks. When JZ started working there, the octopuses got out of the tanks by pushing the lids aside. They got out into the street. There was a headline in a local paper, 'English Professor Teaches Octopuses to Speak'. Five of us worked on octopuses and one, me, on squids.

The following quote from JZ's book, A Model of the Brain, will help me explain the nature of the research that was undertaken on the octopuses.[3]

> 'In the search for food an octopus uses as mainly its many eyes and the receptors in the arms for touch and for chemical conditions. Having no shell or powerful defence mechanism the animal lives protected in a cranny of the rocks that is its home. From this it puts out an arm to seize crabs or other likely food objects that pass within its reach. If something appears farther away the octopus may emerge from its home, swim forward by means of the jet from its funnel, and seize the moving object with its arms. The prey is then carried back to the home, paralysed by a secretion of the salivary glands, and held by the jaws of the parrot-like beak and broken up by a rasping file, the radula. In this method of life it is clearly important that the animal should attack only those objects that are likely to yield food, and retreat from any that might sting or bite. There are certainly many enemies lying in wait, for it is common to find that one or more of the arms of an octopus is in process of regeneration, having been bitten off at the tip.

---

[3] J.Z. Young. 1964. A Model of the Brain. Oxford Clarendon Press. p. 70.

The octopus's brain therefore makes repeated decisions whether or not to put out an arm, or to swim out, when objects move in its visual field or are touched by the arms. Recognition of what is suitable to be attacked depends not on an inherited built-in system, but on learning by 'experience' whether attack at a given object is likely to produce food or a painful stimulus.'

The students had a programme to train the octopuses. The quote above demonstrates that octopuses can see and feel and can either attack or retreat or stay 'at home'. A triangle on the end of a rod was dipped into the tank at the same time as a small crab tied to some string. The octopus attacked and ate the crab. This was repeated a number of times until the octopus would attack the triangle alone. It had remembered that the triangle was associated with food. After this was fixed in its memory, JZ would take the octopus, anaesthetise it, and remove a part of its brain. The octopus was returned to its tank and the programme repeated to see whether it had forgotten what it had learnt. If it had forgotten, then that bit of brain removed was part of the memory system. This programme was repeated (with a triangle or other shape) on a fresh octopus, but instead of a crab a small electric shock was given and octopus did not move or retreated. Experiments like this were done using rough and smooth balls so memory associated with touch and feeling could be explored. These experiments had been going on there for decades. One of my student colleagues, Brian Barbier, was tasked to dissect a dead octopus and using a particular dye search for a nerve that JZ thought must exist. After a couple of weeks, he found it. This was my first experience of the excitement of a scientific discovery.

I was the squid man. Each morning, a fisherman would bring in a couple of squids and put them in a tank of sea water near to where I was working. A. L. Hodgkin and A. F. Huxley developed a mathematical model to explain nerve conduction in a giant nerve of squid in 1952. The experiment was to prove the Hodgkin—Huxley formula that the speed of nerve conduction was related to the square root of the diameter of the giant nerve.

The formula is as follows:

$$cv = sqrt(Ka/2R\_2Cm)$$ cv: conduction velocity
K: 10,470 a: radius of axis cylinder
R_2: specific resistance of axoplasm (35.4 Ohms)
Cm: capacity per unit of area of membrane (10^{-6})

JZ taught me what I had to do. A squid was fished out of the tank and its head cut off. The head had the tentacles and continued to move about on the floor for quite a while. This upset me. I then had to open the body of the squid and under a microscope dissect out an axon (nerve). This was done under salt solution to keep the nerve working. Cotton was tied to each end of the nerve, and it was transported a long way across the building to an oscilloscope. An electrical stimulus was applied to one end and the time for this impulse to reach the other end was measured and recorded. The diameter of the nerve was measured and the result put on a graph. The graph and results from previous years were in a tatty exercise book. JZ could dissect out a nerve and keep it alive every time he did the operation. If you input J. Z. Young in Youtube or Wikipedia, there is a video of him dissecting a squid with a commentary.

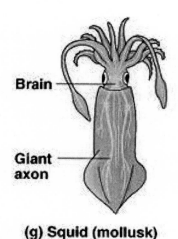

Brain

Giant axon

(g) Squid (mollusk)

The nerves of a squid

It looked so easy. I did this each morning and again in our second work session in the afternoon/early evening. I got no result for three weeks and then I had a success. The reason for not getting a result was that I had been too slow or had damaged the nerve with my dissection. For the second three weeks, I obtained two results each day.

We had a fantastic experience in Naples. We were housed

in apartments. There were three of us in ours. We had breakfast in typical Italian style. We went to a bar and had a cappuccino and a pastry. We started work at 8 a.m. and finished at 12 noon. There was then a four-hour break (siesta) when Italians would go home and rest from the heat. Not us. On many afternoons, JZ would take us off to somewhere like Pompei or Herculaneum. On others, we would do our own thing. We went swimming in the afternoons and I enjoyed snorkelling and diving. There was an underwater Roman ruin about six feet below the surface. We dived and found Roman artefacts such as a piece of a vessel or plate. One time I jumped out of my skin when an octopus emerged from its cranny! We sometimes went swimming at night to see the thousands of small luminous marine organisms that sometimes were present. We went back to work at 4 p.m. and stopped at 8 p.m. We then went out for a meal. Eating and drinking were cheap. There was a fantastic pizzeria with a classical stone oven where we ate outside and drank lots of wine. There was one place nicknamed 'the chicken run'. Chickens would be moving about on the floor of the trattoria. You could choose one and it was then slaughtered and cooked.

One night I drank far too much of the aniseed-based liqueur ouzo and I vomited on the marble floor in our apartment. We cleaned it up but the smell of aniseed remained for several days. How disgusting!

JZ sometimes lent us his car, an estate car, to use in the evenings. We used to drive it too fast and one evening did the Amalfi run, which was a very tortuous but beautiful coastal route. Occasionally, JZ would treat us to a meal in his favourite restaurant. When we arrived, the small orchestra struck up JZ's favourite tune—'Come back to Sorrento'. He had been going there for the past twenty years or so. One evening we went to the laboratory and got an octopus out of its tank. I did not realise how difficult it was to detach eight legs from my arm. We also fooled around wearing JZ's black lab coat.

JZ allowed two of us at a time to have a two-day break. He gave us money. I went with Dave Bromham to Sicily and we stayed one night in the waiting room of Palermo railway station.

When it was time to go back to the UK, JZ asked whether I would drive his car home with some equipment and three of my fellow students. We arrived at the UK customs at about 2 a.m. When asked whether we had anything to declare, I made a big mistake. I said we had an automatic octopus feeding device. I thought the customs officer would laugh and wave us through. He never even smiled. The officer made us unpack the car and show him the apparatus. I was not popular with my friends as we were exhausted.

I found the examination for the B.Sc. difficult. One paper involved writing an essay for three hours. There was a practical examination, and the first thing we had to do was to dissect out the nerve plexus of a pigeon's armpit (the brachial plexus) and write up how it compared with the human brachial plexus. Fortunately, we had found out the previous day that this was coming up. The main difference was that the nerve to the pectoralis major muscle (chest) in a pigeon was huge because this muscle is used to flap its wings. At the London, they had to dissect out the muscles of a monkey's leg and label each one.

We met in a pub to receive our results from JZ. Four of us got firsts, four upper seconds, and four, including me, lower seconds. He told me he had fought at the examiner's meeting for me to be awarded an upper second but failed. I was happy with the lower second. Robin Harrod came top of all thirty anatomy B.Sc. students in the University of London. Robert Tresman came second. Robert had such poor writing that his papers were sent to the London University deciphering unit to be typed out.

The exams and results were at the end of summer term, and I was due to start my clinical studies after the summer holiday in September. My friends were already eighteen months into their studies at University College, and I would have normally followed them. However, earlier in the term, JZ told us he could get us into any teaching hospital in the UK and we could choose. He certainly had some power. One or two opted for the Radcliffe in Oxford, and I opted for the London Hospital, which had turned me down originally. I got an interview with the same dean, Dr John Ellis, as in the first interview. He asked me whether I was intending marrying one of his nurses. I said no and I was accepted immediately. I would be joining my friends Colin Teasdale, Robin Harrod, and Adrian Bomford there.

Of course, all was not work and no play. I mentioned in the last chapter that six of us lived in a flat in Russell Road near Olympia. Let me describe my flatmates in more detail.

Colin Teasdale came to my school in the sixth form. His father was the headmaster of a school in Altofts, West Yorkshire, and they were brought up as Plymouth brethren. Colin has a brother and a sister (who died not so long ago), the former also becoming a doctor as did Colin's son. Colin married Ann, who was a nurse at the London Hospital. It looks as though this could be the start of a medical dynasty. Colin was very fit and was a cross-country runner when we were at school. Colin became a consultant surgeon specialising in breast surgery.

Jim Smeeton I mentioned in Chapter 2. He had a vintage open-topped red MG. He lent it me one weekend to take a friend, Jenny Holgate, to a party in Cheltenham. The party was in the house of a family called Lear. When I started at the London Hospital, the intake was joined by students who had done the part one at Cambridge. One of these was Roger Lear and we became friends. It was his house where the Cheltenham party was held. I see him every year at a reunion that some of us go to. Jim loved sailing, and the only time I have been sailing was with him on Hyde Park Lake in London. We were becalmed for over an hour. Jim became a GP. He passed away not so many years ago and is sadly missed by his friends.

Grahame Smith came from Hereford. Some of us visited and stayed with his parents. Grahame became a GP in Pontefract, which is four miles from where I live in Castleford. He was my GP and I his.

Colin Parker came from the midlands and had a great laugh. It must have been awful to fail second MB with all your friends passing and moving on. He became a GP.

Steve Haggie was from Bedfordshire. He became a surgeon in Rotherham.

It was in that flat I had my first and only fist fight. It was one Saturday afternoon, and I was in the sitting room by myself listening to a gramophone record of Beethoven. Colin came in and switched it off and turned on the TV to watch sport. I was really angry and laid into him. Jim poured some water over us to stop it.

We had few arguments, but one was about whose turn it was to do the washing up of the dishes. This resulted in no one doing the washing up and every single piece of cutlery, crockery, cooking utensils, and so on, piled up in the sink.

Several of us had cars. One game was to put the car keys on the coffee table and on the word 'go', we had a race to Leicester Square and back for some silly prize.

We had read about water intoxication. We did not know that this was potentially fatal and that the majority of deaths were from water drinking competitions. On one occasion, we tried to get drunk on drinking lots of pints of water. I don't think anything happened.

I did an experiment on myself with alcohol. I was alone in the flat. I bought two bottles of red wine from different vineyards situated in the same valley. I wanted to train my palate to tell the difference between the two. I wrote notes as I went along. I had got well down each bottle when one of the flatmates came in and substituted my glass with one containing the liquid from a jar of pickled beetroot. I was so inebriated that I did not notice for a second or two.

During this time, I started to go out with my now wife, Kathleen, and we had a wonderful time together. We got to know one another's parents and went on holiday to Scotland with mine. We split up soon after I started my clinical training.

CHAPTER 4

CLINICAL MEDICAL STUDENT

The London Hospital is situated in the heart of the East End of London on the Whitechapel Road. The London Hospital Medical College was in Turner Street, and there was a back door that opened into a courtyard of the hospital. There was also a tunnel between the medical college building and the hospital. At the end of the tunnel was a shop where I bought my cigarettes. When I walked in, the shop assistant immediately reached out for a packet of Rothmans without my saying anything. This was bad! In the medical school building, in the 1960s, there were the preclinical departments of anatomy, physiology, and biochemistry as well as the dean's office and administration offices.

I have obtained most of the historical material about the London Hospital and its medical college from Sir John Ellis's book.[4] Dr John Ellis was the dean for most of my time at the London.

The London hospital opened on 27 October 1785, four years before the start of the French Revolution. It is a teaching hospital of the highest order. It is also a fine research establishment. In the past, there have been some remarkable innovations made there: James Parkinson—Parkinson's disease, 1817; Thomas Barnado—Dr Barnado

---

[4]   LHMC 1785-1985. 1986. *The Story of England's First Medical School.* Sir John Ellis. London Hospital Medical Club.

children's homes; Sir Harry Souttar—the first to open a chamber of the heart. Sir Frederick Treves was the surgeon who discovered, looked after, and investigated the 'Elephant man', John Merrick in the 1880s. John Merrick had a rare bone growth disease. The film of the story of the elephant man was made in 1980 and starred John Hurt as John Merrick and Anthony Hopkins as Frederick Treves.

In 2009, a BBC series called *Casualty 1909* starring Cherie Lunghi captures the horrific medical and social problems that were dealt with in the East End of London at the beginning of the twentieth century.

When I started there as a clinical medical student in 1966, the East End of London was a significantly deprived area with mainly Jewish and Bangladeshi residents. There were tramps sitting on the pavements. The favourite drink of the tramp was methylated spirits. There was a hostel for the homeless. Reginald and Ronald Kray (the Kray twins) ran

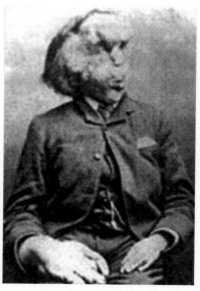

John Merrick

a criminal gang based around Whitechapel. They frequented a pub, The Blind Beggar, which was directly opposite to the London Hospital. We never went into that pub in the evenings. It was far too dangerous.

The hospital was granted a Royal Title by the Queen in 1990. From that time it was known as The Royal London Hospital.

In recent years, there has been a huge building programme, and when completed, the Royal London will be the biggest hospital in Europe.

I started as a clinical student there in the autumn. The B.Sc. students like me were joined by those from Oxford and Cambridge who had also taken three years to get to this point. We were also joined by those who had had to resit the second MB examination. Mike Dawson and Sylvester Kumar were two of these and we became close friends.

We started with a twelve-week introductory course. This was the brainchild of professor of medicine, Clifford Wilson. There were lectures, demonstrations, ward work, and eventually dealing with a real patient. We started studying pathology for which there was an examination at the end of the first year.

The textbook that was a must for this course was the book *Hutchinson's Clinical Methods* by Donald Hunter and R. R. Bomford. This was very much written and edited by London Hospital men. Bomford and Hunter were physicians (Bomford was working at the hospital at the time but Hunter had retired) and Sir Robert Hutchinson became president of the Royal College of Physicians. The book was last published in 2007, and I hope there will be further editions.

The book and the course enabled us, in a very basic way, to start to be able to listen to patients' problems, talk to them, examine them, and decide on possible diagnoses. It must have been a daunting task for the teachers on that course to get us to a point where we were trusted to be with ill and worried people. It was daunting for me too. There was a huge mountain to climb for me.

We were taught a formal way of recording the patient's story (history) and background. Most of this came from questioning the patient but some from the medical records. One focussed on the patient's occupation, social background, and history of the presenting problem, past medical history, family history, medication, smoking, and alcohol. Direct questions were asked about the presenting problem. If, for example, the patient said he was going to the lavatory to pass urine too many times, the following questions would be asked. Was there any blood in the urine? How many times does the patient get up in the night to pass urine? Is there any pain? Is there a good flow?

Working on improving my consultation skills continued until I retired as a GP as I will describe in a later chapter. It is the crux of being a decent doctor. Let me give one example of what we were taught about how to listen to the patient and observe body language. How a patient describes a pain can give a strong clue as to the diagnosis. A chest pain might be described as 'crushing' or 'like someone pressing on my chest' and accompanied by the patient squeezing his hands together. This could be a heart attack or angina.

There was also a formal way of examining a patient. We knew how to take a blood pressure from our physiology teaching but that was about it. We started to learn to look at the patient and observe how he or she walked, the facial expression, the build of the body, and the mental state. I realised that even taking the pulse was not straightforward. The pulse could be regular or irregular, bounding or flat, again clues to a diagnosis.

Generally, for each area of the body, there was a routine approach for the examination: observation (looking), auscultation (listening), percussion (tapping), and palpation (feeling). This routine particularly suits the examination of the chest or abdomen.

I will give the chest as an example. Observation would include the shape, the rate of breathing, the colour, and state of the skin.

Auscultation is listening with a stethoscope. This was very difficult to learn other than examining as many patients as possible. You might hear no sounds of breathing over one lung or part of a lung. You might hear exaggerated sounds. What you heard would contribute to a diagnosis.

Percussion involves tapping a finger of one hand placed on the chest with a finger of the other hand to determine what is underneath. This was really difficult to learn. My flatmates and I practised on one another in the evenings. We were told that it was possible to find where a coin was under a telephone directory using percussion and we tried this. I think someone was joking.

Palpation means feeling with the hands a lump or the trachea (wind pipe) deviated to one side in the front of the neck.

I don't wish this to be a text book of medicine but to give an impression of the vast learning that a medical student has to undertake to be able to crudely assess a patient after twelve weeks.

The introductory course and *Hutchinson's Clinical Methods* taught us to be able to examine every part of the body as well as take a history from a patient. This preparatory learning looked at each of the body's systems, for example, respiratory, gastrointestinal, nervous, and so on, as well as more specific areas such as eyes, blood diseases, ear, nose, and throat, and trauma. Specimen and blood collection and interpreting the results were part of the pathology course.

We had to spend a day in the role of a nurse on one of the wards. This made me empathise with the nurses and realise what an awful part of their job it was to empty and sterilise bedpans. The nurses' uniforms at the London Hospital were unique and certainly did not reflect the clothing revolution that took place in the 1960s.

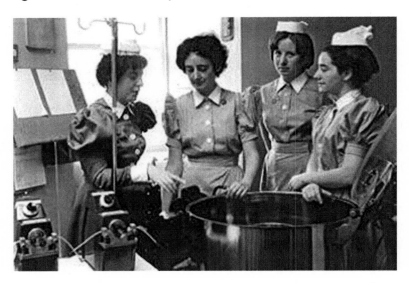

Nurses learning about the intensive therapy unit in 1967[5]

---

5   Courtesy of The Royal London Hospital Archives

Not so long before I started at the London, first thing every morning, the sister of a ward would lead prayers with her nurses kneeling.

I must be a rare medical student in that I never dated a nurse. When I was fifty-five years old, I did take out our practice nurse, Jackie Spencer, for a lunch provided by Huddersfield University relating to the nurse practitioner course she was undertaking. I was her supervisor.

We learnt how to examine the back of an eye with an ophthalmoscope. I actually never mastered this fully the whole of my medical career. We were taught how to take a blood sample from a patient. Listening for abnormal heart sounds such as clicks and murmurs was a challenge. This course certainly made me appreciate the work my parents were undertaking as GPs.

The time arrived when I was to take the history and examine my very first patient. She was a good-looking ballet dancer in her mid-twenties. The problem was that she kept passing out and a provisional diagnosis of attacks of hypoglycaemia (low blood sugar) had been made. I was so nervous and embarrassed such that when I examined her that a drop of sweat fell from the tip of my nose on to her abdomen.

During the introductory course, we had a tutor. The four anatomy B.Sc. students in our year were Adrian Bomford (the nephew of R. R. Bomford, the co-author of *Clinical Methods*), Robin Harrod, Colin Teasdale—my friend from school—and me. We were given a tutor who was a surgeon—Mr Grant-Williams. We met at his house and the subjects for the tutorials were very general. Only Adrian did not have a Yorkshire accent, and on one occasion, Grant—Williams advised us to have elocution lessons. He told us we would never get on in the field of medicine if we continued to talk like we did. He came from Liverpool and had had such lessons. We took absolutely no notice and my Yorkshire accent became more pronounced, I am sure.

One thing seriously disturbed me shortly after I started as a clinical student. The B.Sc. course had a culture of being able to question anything and of mutual respect between teacher and student. Some of the consultant teachers frightened us to death and gave the impression they were always right. These consultants did not encourage questioning. They were eminent indeed but thought they were Gods. One consultant was so horrible to David McGiven that sweat appeared on his back having passed through his shirt, jumper, and white coat.

We lived in several flats during the three-year clinical study time. We gave up the flat in Russell Road and my University College flatmates went their own way with accommodation. Two school friends who had completed their Cambridge degrees joined us in a flat in Walthamstow. Peter Garlick, a school friend, was doing research at St Mary's Hospital. Ian McNeil, another friend from the Wakefield school, was studying medicine at Guys Hospital also lived there. Sylvester Kumar joined us. He was half Bolivian and half English and came from Peru. After that, I lived in a flat in Clapham followed by Tower Hamlets and then a flat in a tower block in Maida Vale.

The flat in Buckmaster Road, Clapham, was very basic. At one point, we had two televisions neither of which worked properly. One TV received sound and the screen flashed on and off. We covered that one with a raincoat and watched the other, which could not receive sound but had a decent black and white picture. The flat was the first floor of a semi-detached house, and when it rained, the roof leaked such that we had to use buckets and pans to collect the drips. In the flat below lived an elderly man called Jack. Social services delivered his lunch every day (meals on wheels). He was perfectly capable of shopping and cooking, which he did, throwing out the meal that had been delivered. One time when Sylvester was particularly hard up, he asked Jack whether he could have his meals on wheels. Jack was the uncle of one of the 'Great Train Robbers' and had an unopened letter addressed to him. There was no way Jack was going to had this over to the police. He would keep it until his nephew came out of prison.

The flat in Tower Hamlets was essentially for one person with a living room cum kitchen, bathroom and a bedroom. Three of us took it on—Colin Teasdale, Kevin Pavey, and myself—and this resulted in the rent being very affordable. The bedroom was very cramped and each of us had their own alarm clock the ticking of which drove Kevin mad. One morning, the other two had gone out and I was in bed. A lorry crashed into the wall of the flat and bricks were dislodged beneath my bed. When I left that flat, my place was taken by Brian Colvin (later to become a consultant haematologist and a dean at the London Hospital). Many years later, when I was a GP, I attended a postgraduate education course he was running. He mentioned me in his introduction. When he took over my bed in Tower Hamlets flat, he found loads of my shoes under it. He referred to me as 'The Imelda Marcos of Whitechapel'. (The Marikina City Footwear Museum in Manila has an exhibition of her shoes. She was the first lady of the Philippines.)

The flat in Maida Vale was luxurious. Again it was basically a flat for a couple with a double bedroom that opened with a sliding door to the living room off which was a kitchen. I think, at one time David Frost had an apartment in that tower block. The flat was on the ninth floor, and I shared with Sylvester Kumar, who slept in the living room. I was the official tenant. One weekend he left the bath running, and it flooded over and leaked down through all nine floors. Fortunately, there was not much damage. We were approaching the final examination, and I wanted to do some significant work. I think Sylvester was still on Peruvian time. He slept in a lot and was not doing much work, and he infected me somewhat. I was frightened we would both fail our exams. He was a seriously nice, good, and kind person, and I felt really guilty when I asked him to leave. He moved in with Adrian Bomford in a flat just behind the medical college. Adrian made him get up and work in the library. We both passed.

After the introductory course, we were allowed to form in groups of twelve and we stuck roughly in that group for the rest of the three-year clinical course. We were allocated to what was called a 'firm'. The consultants teaching on my first firm were Dick Bomford, a diabetologist, and John Ellis, a general physician and the dean. We were allocated patients to 'clerk'. Clerking means taking their medical story or history and examining them. We then wrote our findings up in the patient's records. There would be ward rounds with one or other of the consultants (six of us would work with Dr Ellis and six with Dr Bomford for a month or so then swap over). On a ward around, the student had to present the details of his patient to the group and would be asked questions by the consultant. There would also be tutorial sessions in a small teaching room off the ward. Dr Ellis was a smoker (Players Weights), and we were allowed to smoke in his teaching sessions. There was no teaching relating to general practice at all during the three years. I asked Dr Ellis why not. He replied, 'If you want to see general practice, come and see me working on the ward'. All teaching hospitals now have a department of general practice. Dick Bomford was charming, polite, and a great teacher. These attachments to firms were a sort of apprenticeship. They were great learning experiences. There were lectures to attend, and sometimes a patient would be brought to the lecture to demonstrate something. The main lecture theatre was called The Bearsted Lecture Theatre. Viscount Bearsted was the Mayor of London in 1902 and in 1926 paid for the lecture theatre and a research scholarship.

One lecture was particularly dramatic. It was on amputation by the orthopaedic surgeon Sir Reginald Watson Jones. He had a maroon-coloured Rolls Royce car with a chauffeur who dressed in a similar-coloured uniform. He was orthopaedic surgeon to the Queen. At one point during the lecture, he was waving a huge knife about and accidentally cut his leg. He had to be taken to casualty.

The four of us (Colin, Adrian, Robin, and I) were allowed to choose our own tutor for the rest of the clinical studies. We chose Frank Vince mainly because he had a reputation of being tough, and we thought he would be able to keep this somewhat rebellious group in order. He was an expert in hormones and dwarves. He was a senior registrar at that time. He would set us essays to write, and then, after he had marked them, these would be the basis of a tutorial. If we got things wrong, he told us off in no uncertain manner.

We were taught pathology in the first year, and there was an examination at the end of that period. The professor of pathology was Israel Donniach. He was an excellent teacher and an expert in thyroid disease. He did rounds on the wards assessing patients who were going to die in the very near future and who would be having a post-mortem in his department. Of course they were unaware he was a pathologist. At lunchtimes, there would be presentations of post-mortems open to all students. The house officer would start by presenting the clinical history, examination, and investigations. Then the post-mortem result would be presented. It was amazing how many abnormalities were discovered at post-mortem that had not even been dreamed of while the patient was alive. These findings had not necessarily contributed to the death. The first post-mortem teaching session I ever attended was one on a tramp. He was a methylated spirit drinker. He had lit a cigarette, and in the process the meths fumes exploded in his trachea and bronchi, killing him. I can still picture the charred specimen that was held up for us to view. Another post-mortem that was significant to me was one of a man who had died from a cancer of the stomach. The house officer presented all the clinical findings, and when he had finished, Professor Donniach asked what the patient was in the habit of eating. It had not crossed anyone's mind that diet could be a contributing factor to a disease of the stomach.

There were also some forensic pathology lectures. The professor of forensic medicine was Francis Camps, who was famous for his involvement with murders. He gave evidence at the trial of John Christie, who hid many bodies he had killed at 10 Rillington Place. Professor Camps undertook detailed examination of all of these bodies and proved that Timothy Evans had been wrongly executed for this crime.

During one lecture, we were shown a photograph of a corpse's head where the hair had covered up a bullet exit hole. This had been missed by a number of doctors who had examined that body. The man had committed suicide by shooting himself in the roof of the mouth. For the whole of my medical career, whenever I had to examine a dead body, I always looked for a possible bullet hole in the skull.

We had to learn how to look at histology slides of diseased tissues as well as how to interpret blood test results. There was a large pathology museum with a huge collection of specimens. I and my friends all passed the pathology examination at the end of the first year.

As our time with the first firm was drawing to an end, Drs Bomford and Ellis threw a party for us. Mike Dawson had leanings towards communism and, after a few drinks, tried to persuade Dr Ellis to join the communist party. Mike told us that his ambition was to be a consultant and would have an old-fashioned till in his private consulting room into which he would put the patients' fees.

The next firm was surgery. One of the surgeons on that firm was Mr Hermon-Taylor. He was famous having invented the flexible gastroscope that enabled the inside of the stomach to be visualised using a movable tip. He discovered a method of treating perforated stomach ulcers without operating. This was known as the 'suck and drip' technique. The perforation would seal up if the stomach fluids were sucked up by a tube and the patient fed by an intravenous drip. He also showed that it was safe to drain the fluid out of cysts. He was very posh and invited us to the end of firm party in his smart apartment overlooking Regent's Park. His son, John, became a surgeon, eventually becoming Professor at St George's Hospital, London. John dated the actor Dianna Rigg for a time.

As with a medical firm, there were ward rounds, tutorials, patients to clerk, and lectures. There were two tasks we had to undertake in addition to these learning activities.

The first was male students had to shave their male patients in the early evening the day before their surgery. The shaving was from the nipples to the knees. One usually did the shaving in pairs, taking half of the body each. One evening Mike Dawson and I had a bet as to who could shave their half of a patient the fastest. I wonder what that patient thought. The second undertaking was to assist at operations. I never liked this and decided to avoid getting involved with surgery as much as possible. We scrubbed up and put on a mask, gown, and surgical gloves. The consultant would be the main operator, and he would have an assistant or two depending on the complexity of the operation. A theatre sister would be in charge of the instruments, and of course there was an anaesthetist who also might have an experienced assistant or a junior registrar helping. There was sometimes background music playing. The role of the medical student was to suck out blood when requested or cut the suture material after the surgeon had tied a knot. There was one surgeon who shouted at the student after he or she had cut the suture material. He either shouted 'too short!' or 'too long'. It was never right. One student, at the start of an operation, asked him: 'How would you like the sutures cut, Sir? Too long or too short?' We had to assist at operations once or twice a week. The operation was performed on the patient we had clerked, and we followed up their progress after they returned to the ward. Getting to see a patient from their admission to their discharge after an operation was a great learning experience and a great opportunity to learn how to establish a professional relationship and communicate with patients.

In the three years of clinical studies, I was attached to two or three surgical firms for varying lengths of time. One was the firm of Tresidder and Blandy. They were urosurgeons. Gerald Tresidder was a great communicator, and we regularly attended his outpatients during which a dozen or so men were on couches in cubicles with their legs splayed apart and held in stirrups. They were all waiting to have an examination of the bladder (cystoscopy).

These cystoscopies were not done under general anaesthetic. A local anaesthetic gel was introduced into the urethra of the penis, and after it had acted, the bladder was examined with a cystoscope. The whole thing looked excruciatingly painful to me. However, pain is often in the eye of the beholder. These clinics were usually held in the morning, and halfway through, the sister would announce that Dr Broadbent had arrived. For two or three weeks, I could not identify which person was Dr Broadbent. Then I realised. They were the code words for the coffee break.

Prof. John Blandy was a great cartoonist as well as a painter and sculptor. He was an expert in testicular cancer and prostates as well as other areas of urology. At that time, I had the idea to investigate the fact that when one kidney is removed from the body, the other enlarges despite a human requiring only part of one kidney to survive. How did one kidney 'know' when the other had been removed? There must have been some hormone or chemical involved. What was the point of it? Peter Garlick was researching on rats at St Mary's Hospital in Paddington. He supervised my operating on a couple of rats. I took one kidney out. I weighed the kidney I had taken out and then the other after the rat had been killed humanely after a few weeks. These were the only animal experiments I ever undertook. I told Professor Blandy of my interest and he lent me an instrument for measuring kidneys on X-rays. He arranged for X-rays before and after nephrectomy operations to be put out for me, and I measured the kidneys. I did this in the early evenings. I did not get anywhere, but I thought it was great to be encouraged like that.

Another firm I worked on had a vascular surgeon, Douglas Eadie, as one of the surgeons. He was a little bit frightening. In the last six months of my clinical studies, I wrote an article for the London Hospital Gazette entitled '10 steps to getting a house job at The London'. It was meant to be humorous, and I wrote about how many paces behind a consultant one should walk and how to butter them up generally. I heard that Mr Eadie had said during an operation that I would never get a house job with him. I panicked that I had ruined my career but all turned out well in the end. Mr Eadie did one of the first aortic and upper femoral artery replacements with artificial material. It was a huge operation and took many hours and everybody in the hospital knew it was going on. Unfortunately, the patient died after the operation and his artificial arteries are preserved as a pathology specimen in the museum.

Another even more formidable surgeon who taught us was Charles (Charlie) Mann. He was also a finals examiner as well as an editor of a standard surgical textbook, Bailey and Love. He was a colorectal surgeon. He had the habit of shouting at you if you got something wrong. He once asked a group of us what we should examine in a patient who complained of weight loss. I answered, 'the anus, Sir.' He bellowed, 'Balls'. I replied, 'No, I wouldn't examine them. Sir'. Everyone in the group laughed, but Charlie Mann's face looked thunderous. He did the jokes. To my horror, he was the viva examiner for surgery finals. I was petrified. However, he came out of his room, put his arm around my shoulders, and was charming throughout the viva examination, which I passed. My mother's cousin, Klaus Turner, lived in London and had a rectal bleed. He ended up in the London under the care of Charlie Mann, who performed a colostomy. I met Mr Mann in the quadrangle outside the medical school and asked him how my relation was. He replied that he could not talk about him as that would have been a breach of confidentiality. However, he said, 'When I do an operation of this type, it always results in a cure'. My relation was indeed cured and lived a long life after that.

I will continue to write about our clinical teaching after I have described some of our recreational activities as students of the 1960s. I mentioned in Chapter 2 that I went out with Kath until the early part of my clinical studies. We decided we should end our relationship, and I then went out with Felicity Sutton, a medical student at St Mary's hospital, who lived in the same hall of residence as Kath. We married shortly after I completed my house jobs.

I never heard of anyone or saw anyone take drugs or smoke pot. However, there was certainly very significant drinking of alcohol by most of us.

I was alone in the flat one evening when Colin arrived back and announced to me, 'You have been elected. You are in'. I did not know what he was talking about. I was elected to the Dionysian's Society. Dionysus was the Greek god of the grape harvest, winemaking, and wine, and the society was a drinking club. Colin took me to the Good Samaritan pub, which was next door to the college clubs union. There were many members of the society there, and it was about 9 p.m. I was bought several pints of beer by pub closing time at 11 p.m. I was very merry indeed. I was then told there was a task I had to undertake before I was admitted as a member of the society. The task was to drink a yard of beer without taking my lips away from it.

That night the pub had no yard but there was a boot. The boot contained three pints, slightly more than a yard. The rule was that one had to continue drinking even if one vomited. I managed it without being sick during the drinking. The society met every Wednesday evening and had its own tie. This must be worn all day each Wednesday. If a member was found not wearing his tie had to pay for the drinks in the pub that night. I did forget my tie once and locked myself in a study room for the day. The society has an annual dinner. I went to one in the very early days. The dinner was usually very rowdy and sometimes damage was caused to the venue resulting in the society being banned. The reservation for the dinner was made once in the name of the London Hospital Christian Union.

There were debates held in the student (Clubs) union. One debate had the motion 'that this house believes that humour is the best medicine'. One of the speakers was a student senior to me called Bob Winston (now the eminent expert in fertility, broadcaster, and author, Lord Robert Winston). Another speaker was the consultant neurologist, Ronald Henson. (We used to call his teaching sessions 'Henson's Half Hour' after the comedian Tony Hancock's TV programme, Hancock's Half Hour.) The two other speakers were the well-known comedians Charlie Chester and Cardew Robinson. The debate was great fun and I wrote the report of it in the London Hospital Gazette.

Rugby union was a very serious activity with some excellent players. We supported our hospital in the United Hospitals Challenge Cup. There were six or eight teaching hospitals from London in the competition, which was fierce. The London Hospital Rugby Football Club (RFC) was founded in 1865. Loads of students went to the matches, and there plenty of beer was downed. Brian Colvin was a very good player as was Norman Williams and Danny Ash; Norman was at the time of writing the recently appointed President of the Royal College of Surgeons and Danny Ash became a consultant oncologist at Leeds.

We played cards a lot both in the clubs union and back at our flat. Bridge and poker were the main games. We played poker for money and a whole term's grant money could be lost and the start of a term. We played bridge for hours on end. Attendance at certain teaching sessions was not compulsory, and we missed quite a lot of teaching. I missed nearly a month of gynaecology outpatients teaching and played cards instead. We played all sorts of varieties of poker. One variety was called whores, fours, the one-eyed jacks (jacks of spades and hearts), and the man with the axe (the King of diamonds) wild. The whores were the queens. We sometimes played cards at the back of the room during a lecture.

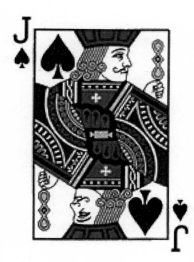

One-eyed Jack

A few of us visited Regents Park Zoo after having been at the pub. Mike Dawson climbed over the fence to save the entrance fee. I was too cowardly to do that but bet Mike a pint of beer that he would not dare to run to the middle of the snake pit and back. I lost the bet.

A huge amount of time went into planning an operation in Trafalgar Square to float helium-filled balloons up Nelson's column and lodge them at the top. Many students were involved, and we even had decoys to distract any policemen. The venture failed as the police noticed we were all wearing white plimsolls, and they caught the balloons just as they were released. None of us got into trouble, and we left with the police loading the balloons into a large van.

Great and close friendships were made during the clinical studies. Some of those on the firm have been meeting for an annual reunion for more than forty years. The present group are Brian Colvin and Kate; Steve Shalet, and Barbara; Graham Hillman and Francine; Colin Teasdale and

Ann; Kevin Pavey and Sheila; Roger Lear and Linda; Robin Harrod and Christine; Mike Dawson and Pauline; Dave Stern and Penny; Kath and I. Anne was a nurse, Christine a dental, and Shelagh a medical student at the London.

There were parties and dances. I had my twenty-first birthday party back in Castleford and lots of friends from London came. We young ones used the surgery rooms that were adjacent to the house. We drank cider and beer. My parents had a few friends over for drinks. Steve Shalet arrived a bit late and entered the room where my parents were entertaining and asked, 'Is there any of the hard stuff?' and then realised his mistake.

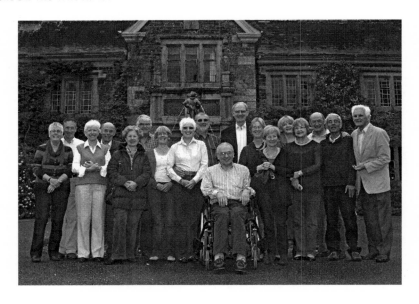

Reunion 2011. From left to right: Penny, Dave, Linda, Roger, Francine, me, Kath, Christine, Robin, Colin, Brian, Shelagh, Ann, Barbara, Kate, Steve, Kevin, Graham

Apart from medicine, pathology, urology, and surgery, there were a daunting number of disciplines to learn about and be able to diagnose and treat: eyes, ear, nose, and throat, venereology, obstetrics, gynaecology, skins, neurology, psychiatry, orthopaedics, family planning, emergencies, therapeutics. I will try and give you a taste of the learning we undertook in some of these areas.

We each had to deliver about twenty babies during our obstetric attachment, and we were in competition with student midwives. Part of this was undertaken at the London and part at an outside hospital. Some of the deliveries were undertaken in flats or houses near to the London Hospital. The first delivery I observed was one of those. The midwife who mainly undertook home deliveries we called Aunty Gladys. There was a bicycle at the front of the hospital for use of the students to get to the patient and one for Aunty Gladys. To my horror, I arrived at the flat and Aunty Gladys was not yet there. It was a slum and the patient was having her fourth or fifth baby. They were a lovely family. The husband said to me, 'Of course you'll need plenty of hot water, Doctor'. I had no idea what the hot water was for. I thought, maybe, it was used to somehow flush out the baby. It turned out that the hot water was for washing our hands. Aunty Gladys arrived, and I watched my first delivery, which was an absolutely marvellous experience for me. While doing obstetrics at the London, the wife of Mr Hartgill, one of the consultant obstetricians, was rushed, in labour, to the hospital (with a police escort). We thought she would have very special treatment. However, they allowed my friend and fellow student John McCardy to deliver her. Mike Dawson and I spent one month living at Oldchurch Hospital, Romford, to complete our obstetric experience. We were supervised doing normal deliveries. Sometimes, if the head of the baby was having difficulty or was expected to have difficulty in the very last stage of labour, an episiotomy was performed. This is an incision using scissors on the posterior vaginal wall to enlarge the opening. The incision was made after local anaesthetic. After the baby and placenta were delivered, the cut had to be stitched up. Sisters were allowed to do episiotomies, and Mike and I were woken nearly every night to stitch these. These days episiotomies are hardly done. In the evenings, we watched TV in the common room, and in the daytime, if things were slack, we each had permission to play the organ in the hospital church. One afternoon the neighbouring gas works were thought to be at risk from an explosion, and we had to evacuate all the women to a distant part of the hospital.

This included women in labour. At the end of the obstetrics training, we had undertaken our twenty normal deliveries and maybe a breech. We had assisted at caesarean section operations. We also learnt how to examine a pregnant woman, how to manage a normal pregnancy, and how to diagnose pregnancy problems. This was my first experience of a hospital away from the London. I realised how much the National Health Service relied on doctors trained overseas. Some evenings we were the only English medics in the hospital. Obstetric training took two months. However, in order to become a GP looking after obstetric cases, one had to undertake further experience in maternity care and then one could register on the 'obstetric list'. I will explain this further in the chapter on general practice.

We spent a number of weeks learning psychiatry. The patients we were allocated were often severely ill. Again some of the learning was undertaken at the London and some at outside hospitals such as St Clements Hospital. St Clements was opened as a workhouse in 1848 and became a hospital for psychiatric patients in 1936. It was closed in 2005. In my time, there were two patients each of whom thought he was Jesus Christ. They used to spit at one another at meal times. I asked one patient of mine to tell me what the problem was and he replied, 'It's obvious, can't you see?' I did not understand, and after several attempts at my guessing, he told me, 'I haven't got a body'. Another patient had the severest of depression after the death of her dog. I asked the head of psychiatry, Prof. Desmond Pond, whether I should write this up in the medical notes that covered housing, job, and finances, and so on—the social history. He told me that pets should be included in the area where are noted details about the medical problems of the patient's family—the family history. Later in my life, as a dog owner and GP, I realised how strong the bond is between owner and a pet.

After preclinical study, then the anatomy degree (three years) and another three years clinical studying the final examination approached. I was a nervous wreck. All the theoretical and practical learning to be tested to see whether one was fit to practise as a doctor.

The examination was a mixture of writing essays, multiple choice questions, and vivas (one-to-one conversations with an examiner). The examination room for the written parts was set out with tables, and there were two students per table. My partner on our table was Janet Share. She was a very bright girl who had done a B.Sc. in Physiology. After a while of us both writing our answers, she whispered to me that I was writing in such a way that I was shaking the table. This created serious anxiety for me, but I somehow changed my writing technique that satisfied her. The final examinations went on for several weeks, and we were exhausted at the end of them.

What a glorious feeling it was to pass that final examination and be a doctor! What a privilege it was to be qualified as a doctor to look forward to curing people, help suffering, and prevent diseases! I felt over the moon to have a title of 'doctor'. This was actually a courtesy title as really only a Ph.D., MD, or D.Sc. were really truly entitled to be called 'doctor'. I became a proper doctor later. I had an MB (Bachelor of Medicine) and BS (Bachelor of Surgery) to add to my B.Sc.

However, my mother pointed out that when one reaches the peak of one stage in one's career, one moves to the very bottom of the next stage. It is also a humbling thought that the word 'degree' can mean a stage in a series of steps in a process. A degree is the start of something not the end.

CHAPTER 5

HOUSE OFFICER

The next stage was a year of house officer jobs at the end of which one became registered with the General Medical Council. That meant one could practice in any branch of medicine. We applied for house officer jobs at the London Hospital and its associated hospitals, but it was by no means certain that everyone would get a job there. It was expected that one undertook a six-month house job in medicine followed by surgery or vice versa. I think the students who did the best in the finals got the best jobs, like Robin who got a medical unit job.

My first house job was a medical one at Mile End Hospital, a short distance away from the London Hospital. I was very nervous. My heart sank when I found out that the senior registrar on that firm was Frank Vince, who had been our tough tutor. However, he taught me well. The ward sister was a remarkable woman who ruled with a rod of iron and yet was compassionate and caring. She taught me more than anyone else what was expected of a medical house officer. The hours were long and exhausting. We worked every other weekend from 9 a.m. Saturday to 5 p.m. Monday and could have been up for hours during the nights. If someone's heart stopped, I was part of the crash team. My bleep would sound for an emergency, and everyone on the team ran to the patient. One patient we started to revive told us 'get off'. He had had enough. I was so exhausted one night that I slept right through one of these cardiac arrest calls.

The two consultants I worked for in the first three months of that job were Dr Barbara Boucher, a diabetologist, and Dr Dolphin, a chest physician. Dr Dolphin had very poor vision and wore glasses with very thick lenses. His ward rounds were very slow, and he had a tendency to start going around the patients again because of his sight problem. He was fantastically skilled at examining a patient's chest and diagnosing small abnormalities. He told me that he wished I was on call all the time with no time off at all and then he would not have to go through what had happened to patients with two housemen.

There was a small ward with geriatric patients. One ninety-year-old was in the habit of falling asleep with a cigarette stuck to his lower lip. Dr Dolphin asked me to tell the patient he should stop smoking. This was because of his health rather than his being a fire risk. I pointed out that it was a bit late at his age to stop. Another of these elderly patients tried to light a cigarette when he was in an oxygen tent. It was a good job he failed as the whole ward could have been blown up.

Another man had been admitted with his knee joints fixed at 90 degrees from sitting day and night in an armchair. Every day I had to give him an injection of Valium to render him nearly unconscious. This relaxed his muscles. I then extended his knees a little and fixed the joints in plaster of Paris. I'm not sure all this did any good.

There was an influenza epidemic in the winter of 1969/70. The virus was influenza A2 1968 (Hong Kong). I started this job in the autumn of 1969. As the winter progressed, there were more and more medical admissions with complications of influenza. I felt that my job was to get to new admissions, do a brief examination before he or she died shortly afterwards. I was then able to issue a death certificate. I became really depressed about this situation and indeed was in tears on several occasions. Throughout my training, I was looking forward to helping ill people, and this was not what was happening at all. At night, I was woken by the noise of dead bodies being wheeled to the mortuary. By the end of that six-month job, the flu epidemic had calmed down and so had I.

On occasions at night, one had to be on call for the wards and casualty at the same time. This was manageable with a medical job, which slackened off in the evenings but very awkward for those doing a surgical job, which involved assisting in the operating theatre. Casualty was generally not very busy at night.

Although the hours were long, there were not the investigative facilities available to today's house officers and so, in my opinion, our job was easier then than today.

There was no intensive care unit and heart attacks were admitted to the general medical ward. There were about half a dozen cardiac monitors and often a monitor had to be removed from one patient to be used on a new admission.

The process of learning about a case started with the registrar seeing the patient first, usually in the casualty department. He wrote a brief note with possible diagnoses. I then took over and took details, wrote everything up, and ordered investigations. Towards the end of the job, I asked the registrar not to put the diagnosis down so I could work things out for myself.

The senior registrar, Frank Vince, occasionally met me before he had to go up the road to the London Hospital. On one such occasion, he asked a nurse to bring me the dental instrument tray. This had a vast array of tools I had never seen before. He asked me to remove an incisor tooth from an elderly lady and then left the ward and me holding the dental tray. Fortunately, I could have removed the tooth with my fingers, it was so loose. I think Frank Vince enjoyed putting the fear of God into me. On another occasion, he asked me to do a sigmoidoscopy (examination of the lower bowel with a long metal instrument) on a woman with a deformed spine. Again he left me to it. A nurse showed me what to do, but I found it impossible to carry out. The third episode I remember was his telling me to teach a nurse how to remove blood from an artery. This is quite a dangerous procedure. I had never done it before and went to my bedroom to look it up in a text book. Fortunately, all went OK. Other procedures we were taught were lumbar punctures; draining fluid from the chest (aspiration of a pleural effusion) and abdomen (aspiration of ascites).

The consultants for the second three months were Prof. Mike Floyer (who later became the dean) and Barbara Boucher's husband, Dr R. D. Cohen.

A memorable case taught us all about thinking of rare causes of disease. A woman of about forty years of age who was admitted with retention of urine. She was relieved by a catheter being inserted but each time the catheter was removed, she went into retention again. Loads of investigations were undertaken and nothing came up. Everyone was foxed. It was decided to call in Professor Blandy, the urosurgeon.

He did not examine the patient and told us to prepare her for operation the next morning as she had carcinoma of the cervix. He was proved to be right, and the cancer was extensive and the reason the urine outflow was being blocked. None of us had examined the vagina. She died a few days later. Professor Blandy came to see her, and I had forgotten to tell him she had died. She was in a single room and Professor Blandy was absolutely shocked when he went in and found her covered in a shroud. He really told me off and quite rightly so. Retention of urine is rare in a woman and so is a large carcinoma of the cervix.

At the end of that job, I felt more confident that I could deal with any medical cases that presented in my next six-month job, house officer to the receiving room back at the London Hospital.

The receiving room is so called because it is the department that 'receives' the patients into the hospital. All admissions pass through it, and it is also the accident and emergency (A & E) department (then called casualty). Sir Jon Ellis's book quotes Frederick Treves's description of the receiving room of the late nineteenth century: 'strange scenes, some pathetic, some merely sordid, together with fragments of tragedy in which the most elemental passions and emotions of humanity are displayed'. There were similarities when I worked there in 1970. We met the fantastic spectrum of people who lived in the East End of London. They were cockneys, Jews, and Bangladeshis. It was a deprived area with methylated spirit drinking tramps and vagrants. It could be a violent place with shootings and knife attacks.

Until 1885, the receiving room was manned by the duty surgical or medical house officers who were called to the department by the nurses manning it. Receiving room officers were established that year. There were several receiving room officers working alongside me. We worked in shifts. Later, working as a GP, I could empathise with the coal miners and other shift workers. I had to take a sleeping tablet after I came off a night shift. There were about four senior receiving room housemen, and a consultant orthopaedic surgeon, who was never to be seen, was head of department. One of the sisters in charge was the niece of Professor Cross, the head of the physiology department, where I was to work next. Sister Cross managed the department in a most efficient manner. She had a wicked sense of humour and teased me mercilessly. The receiving room described by Sir Frederick Treves was filthy. The one I worked in was maintained spotless not only by the cleaners but also by the nurses.

The cases we dealt with in the receiving room were a great preparation for general practice. This job was regarded as a surgical house officer appointment. This pleased me as I hated being in an operating theatre. It seems a bit of a farce that I have a degree in surgery, namely Bachelor of Surgery.

I was supervised stitching up a small wound. The first big wound I stitched on my own was on a man's leg that required between twenty and thirty sutures. He came back the next day and 75 per cent of them had come undone.

One week I made a note of all the cases that attended the receiving room. These included nose bleeds, overdoses, head injuries, hypoglycaemic comas, drunks, epileptic fits, burns, strokes, heart attacks, assaults, toothache, hysteria, depression, wax in the ear, migraines, sudden blindness, menstrual problems, wanting to use the lavatory, and so on. The list could go on. These were as well as planned surgical and medical admissions that went through the receiving room. There was a rush of people coming in when the GP's surgeries closed in the evenings. There was a supply of rude letters telling off the GPs and signed by the head of department that we could use.

At night there was just one receiving room officer and a staff nurse working, which was rather cosy when it was not busy. However, we were also on call for any disturbances on the ward. I had one call to the orthopaedic ward where a man was running amok dragging his drip feed around and being generally threatening. He was an alcoholic and had been withdrawn too rapidly from his alcohol. He had delirium tremens. I sorted him out with some sedative. The orthopaedic house officer at the time was my friend Brian Colvin. He told me that he was not called out of bed once while doing that job. What a lucky person!

At night, the rule was that if more than twenty people were in the receiving room, one was allowed to call for extra medical help. One night, eighteen firemen were brought in overcome by heat and fumes, and I had to deal with them all with the help of my nurse colleague. Fortunately, plenty of water to drink and a rest was the cure.

The receiving room officer had to interpret and report on any X-rays taken at night. They were later reported on by a radiologist. We had only had very basic training in how to interpret X-rays. I missed a fractured skull, but fortunately there were no consequences of this.

I gained huge experience during the day shifts. Assaults on Asians were rife in the East End of London at that time. This was verbal as well as physical abuse by non-Asians. The non-Asians were occasionally policemen. The division of the police responsible for the East End were really tough. There was an annual pretty violent game of rugby union between the hospital and police teams. Twenty-four hours a day, we could call a police officer who constantly patrolled the hospital and its grounds.

When a diabetic's blood sugar falls, there is sometimes a period of confusion before he or she becomes comatose if glucose is not administered. The confusion stage can be misdiagnosed as I did with a young woman who wandered in and whom I thought was hysterical. Someone thought of giving her a sugary drink. She was immediately cured and told us she was diabetic. On another occasion, a GP had sent in a man accompanied by a letter stating that he had had a stroke. I checked him over and was about to send him to the ward when I thought I would give him a shot of glucose into a vein. Like the young woman, he completely recovered and was a diabetic on insulin. Generally, it can do no harm injecting or swallowing some glucose and so I did so to anyone who had disturbed consciousness. I light-heartedly called this Sloan's rule.

Suicide attempts were very common particularly with teenage girls. We felt like doing nothing but telling them off and sending them home to their mothers. The most common method was a drug overdose. Paracetamol was particularly dangerous as there is a delayed effect of a day or so to fatal liver damage. It was hard to persuade a perfectly well patient that he or she had to be admitted as an emergency.

A young Bangladeshi man who spoke no English came in clutching a bottle of ABC liniment. He had drunk half a bottle and was feeling ill. ABC liniment intended to be rubbed on painful muscles and joints and was dangerous if taken by mouth. It contains aconite, belladonna, and chloroform. I phoned Guys Poison Centre for advice as to his management. An immediate stomach washout was recommended. The hospital had interpreters but we could not find one. We could not explain what we were proposing. He had to be manhandled on to an examination couch and screamed when we forced him to undertake a stomach washout, which undoubtedly saved his life.

There was one middle-aged man who attended several times a week seriously attempting suicide by means of drug overdoses. He was often brought in deeply unconscious and requiring admission. He really meant it. Just before I left the department, the decision was being made as to whether or not he should be allowed to die and then remove his kidneys for transplanting. I never heard what happened. He is the only patient I saw in the receiving room whose name I remember.

There was a notebook called the black book in which was written amusing incidences that had occurred in the receiving room over the years. One was of a woman who presented at reception complaining that she hadn't 'seen a thing' for three months. She was worried she was pregnant. The receptionist directed her to the eye clinic. I wrote one observation in that book. The treatment of a nosebleed that could not be stopped by pressure on the outside of the nose was to pack the nostril with gauze. This came in a narrow strip and often several feet would be crammed into a nostril. This was removed a couple of days later. I was removing such a pack from the nose of a Jewish man who had come with his brother. The brother said, 'I always wondered where you kept your money'.

Once I had to ask another doctor to take over from me because I could not cope. A plump teenager came in with lower abdominal pain. After other questions, I asked 'And what about your periods?' The patient replied, 'What do you mean, periods?' I explained what periods were. The patient was very upset and exclaimed, 'But I am a boy'. I was so embarrassed that I had to leave the cubicle and get someone else to deal with him.

The team of receiving room officers had to do locums for fellow house officers when they took holidays. This work was instead of the receiving room job and was somewhat daunting but great experience. I did two periods of two weeks as a locum. The first one was on the medical unit working for Prof. Jack Ledingham. He was an expert in hypertension and a real stickler for detail. He spent ages with patients. I arrived thinking that lots of investigations had to be undertaken on each patient and ordered every test I could think of on my first case. I had got that aspect of the job and him completely wrong. Professor Ledingham told me off. The senior registrar on that unit was Frank Goodwin, who tragically died from aids several years later. He asked me whether I would like to see him drain some fluid from a patient's chest and I told him I was not interested and that I was going off duty. I obviously had already secured my next job at that point as deference to our seniors was definitely expected by most of them.

The second locum job I did was working on the kidney dialysis unit. The patients had no kidney function and had to come in to hospital periodically to be attached to a machine through which their blood flowed to be cleansed of the impurities normally undertaken by their kidneys. They were waiting for kidney transplants. It was remarkable how much each patient knew about what should be done to them, any complications, and detecting any problems with the dialysis machine. The patients taught me what I should do rather than my superiors in the medical profession. From that job onwards, I listened hard to patients when they told me how they were dealing with their medical problems.

As I have mentioned, I was not keen on surgery. I even managed, in the middle of the receiving room job (which was regarded as a surgical post), to do a month of medical jobs.

Being able to eat properly when working so hard was very important. There was a canteen for the junior medical staff and there were separate eating arrangements for the nurses. The food in the consultants' dining room was superb, and occasionally they would send food that was left over to the junior doctors. There was also the Blizzard Club in the medical college building. (See Chapter 6). Academics could eat there. By that is meant professors, readers, and senior and junior lecturers. A consultant in the hospital was generally at least a senior lecturer of the college and of the University of London. The food in the Blizzard club was not a gastronomic experience like that of the consultants' dining room. The students ate in the canteen in the Clubs Union Building in Stepney Way. Mike Dawson had the same meal for lunch every day for about six years—pie and baked beans. Off duty, eating in the Whitechapel Road area was fun. There were Indian and Chinese restaurants. The Jewish restaurant Blooms was in Brick Lane but closed in the 1990s. A student wrote a booklet called 'The bad food guide', which described some appalling eating places in the East End, some which were dangerous because of the East End criminal element.

We were so busy as house officers that there having a haircut might be neglected. There was a Jewish barber very near the hospital called 'Sid's'. Sid refused to cut my hair on one occasion because I had a boil on my neck. He sent me out saying he would have to sterilise his scissors. Despite my embarrassment, I think he was quite right. Had I learnt nothing after seven years of training?

It was another great feeling to complete one's house jobs and be registered with the General Medical Council as a doctor. That meant one was free to practise as a GP, or as a hospital doctor. We could write prescriptions anywhere that would employ us.

This was the end of my dealing with and meeting patients from the East End of London. I had had a first taste of multiculturalism and ethnic diversity as well as the cockney sense of humour. Years later, I was in a store in Oxford Street and asked the doorman for directions to a department. He had a heavy cockney accent. I asked him where he lived, and it was near the London Hospital. I told him I had trained and worked there and he told me that he had been an inpatient once. He said, 'You know when the consultant comes around and leans over you to examine you?' He took a pen out of his inside pocket. 'Well, this is his pen'.

I would miss the cockney rhyming slang. Examples are 'I am going out with the trouble and strife'—the wife. 'I fell down the apples and pears'—stairs. Of course the one I really appreciate is 'I was on my tod', which means I was alone. This is double cockney slang. James Forman (Tod) Sloan was an American jockey who was very successful towards the end of the nineteenth and start of the twentieth century. He often won by a huge margin and was way in front of the other horses. So the cockney slang thread goes—On my tod; Tod Sloan, on my own'. It is important to come to grips with how patients communicate not only to empathise with them but also to have an efficient consultation.

I went back home to Yorkshire soon after I was registered and suggested to my mother (my father had retired) that I did her surgery while she prepared the evening meal. I never got past the first patient who came in and asked me for the 'black bombers I take me 'ed'. Here I was encountering yet another communication problem just as difficult as cockney slang. I had to leave the surgery and ask my mother to finish. Registering with the GMC was not the completion of something but the start of a new learning experience. I was proud to be a fully registered doctor but at the same time found the situation daunting. How would I ever be competent as a GP?

CHAPTER 6

PHYSIOLOGY

Physiology is a very broad discipline and is the science of how living things work.

I was in a hospital bed when the reader in physiology, Dr W. R. Keatinge[6], interviewed me for the job of lecturer.

In the last two weeks of my first house officer job, I developed a particularly painful recurrence of an infected pilonidal sinus. A pilonidal sinus is a hair growing inwards and is usually situated at the upper part of the cleft between the buttocks. I was due to get married to Felicity in a few weeks. I had done everything in my power to avoid going into hospital, but by that time it was excruciatingly painful to sit down and I was losing sleep. I was admitted to the private wing of the London Hospital

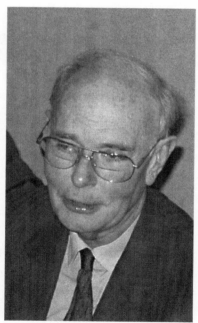

Prof. W. R. Keatinge[6]

6   'Photograph taken by author at a dinner given by Prof. Keatinge held at the Royal Society of Medicine, London.'

(Fielden House). This was a perk for doctors working at the London. I was admitted under a surgeon called Mr Alan Parks, who was eminent in his field of colorectal surgery. (Later: Prof. Sir Alan Parks Kt 1977; PRCS 1980-82; MRCS and FRCS 1949; BA Oxford 1943; BM, BCh 1947; MCh 1954; MD Johns Hopkins 1947; MRCP 1948; FRCP 1976; Hon FRCS Ed 1981; Hon FRCPS Glas 1981; FRCP Ed 1981; FRACS 1981; Hon FRCSC 1982. What a collection of degrees!).

I always maintain that he got his knighthood for operating on me. If one worked on his firm as a student and had achieved performing fifty rectal examinations on patients, one was entitled to buy and wear a special tie—the rectal tie. I think I should be entitled to one having been operated on by him. The operating theatres were in the main building of the London Hospital, which was separate from Fielden House. After I had put on my operation gown and had a pre-medication injection, I was taken to the operating theatre on a trolley. This involved being taken outside and wheeled along a street. It was a good job it was not raining.

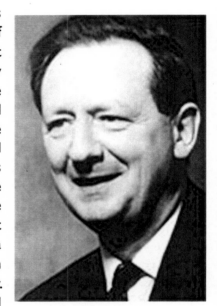

Sir Alan Parks

The house officer who assisted Mr Parks was a houseman from the same year as me, Tony Mathie. He told me that the operation was so major that it had been videoed for training purposes! I believed him for a moment. It was very boring lying about for so long and Tony kindly went to the betting shop almost every day so I could enjoy watching the races on the TV in my room. Tony later became the director of GP Postgraduate Education at the Mersey Deanery and also the treasurer of the Royal College of General Practitioners.

After the operation, I had to lie on my side for about ten days and have the wound packed and dressed regularly. It was a deep and wide wound that healed by tissue building up from its base (healing by granulation). I had to have daily salt baths. In the room opposite was a consultant physician who had had a haemorrhoid (pile) operation. He also had to have daily salt baths. He came to see me with a request: he told me that he was too embarrassed as a consultant to ask the somewhat formidable sister how much salt to put in his bath and he asked me to find out from her. The answer was 'to taste'. When I was allowed to get up a bit I was in the habit, during the night, of looking at my own medical records, which were kept in the corridor. The formidable sister caught me at it and locked them away in her office for the rest of my stay.

The food in Fielden House was superb, and there was a choice from a menu given to patients each morning. I also had a selection of alcoholic drinks at the end of my bed, which I offered to visitors and enjoyed myself. Mr Parks discharged me early one afternoon and complained that I had never offered him a drink. I had ordered trout for my evening meal and did not want to miss that meal. The sister gave me permission to stay in my room until after I had had my supper.

Being a private patient in a London teaching hospital in the late 1960s was certainly an experience for me and would have cost me an absolute fortune if it were not a perk of the job.

I applied for the physiology job because my first wife-to-be, Felicity, was about three years behind me with her medical studies at St Mary's Hospital in Paddington, London. I was interested in research but always intended to be a GP when Felicity had completed her studies. It generally took about three years to undertake research to Ph.D. level.

I was offered the job and was a lecturer in physiology. Help! What had I let myself into?

On the first morning of my job, I arrived in the department at 8.30 a.m. The place was deserted. Bill Keatinge and the head of the department,

Prof. Kenneth Cross, arrived at 9 a.m. and others drifted in as the morning progressed. Some did not come in at all. I realised later that this was part of 'academic freedom'. The technicians worked from nine to five, but the academics could come and go as they pleased. Some of the physiologists had medical degrees. There were also vets, dentists, and others from a variety of scientific backgrounds. I noted that the medics and dentists tended to get in early as this is part of their work ethic. The head of department, Kenneth Cross, was a medic. He once stood at the entrance door of the department and smacked anyone's hand if he or she arrived after 9 a.m.

I had considerable anxieties since I had accepted the job. I was not particularly outstanding at physiology as a student, and it was five-and-a-half years since I did the second MB examination, which included physiology. There had been significant research undertaken in that time and significant advances in the field. It was going to be a steep learning curve for me to be able to undertake original research, lecture to 100 students, and teach in tutorials and practical classes. It was amazing to me that one did not need to have to have had any teaching on educational methods to be a lecturer or a teacher of medical students.

Bill Keatinge showed me to a room I could use and introduced me to people. He told me that I could spend the next three months settling in, preparing lectures, and deciding which physiologist I would ask to be my Ph.D. supervisor. I found this a great luxury. There was some great work going on there and some fascinating and very bright people. There were significant researchers who had studied at Oxford or Cambridge and most had a first-class primary degree. I got a slight inferiority complex with my lower second in anatomy.

In the two laboratories on either side of mine were Fred Smales, who had a dental background, and Jim Barrowman, who was working on an aspect of gastroenterology. Prof. Kenneth Cross was working with David Boulton and Dr Goodwin on cot deaths. Mike Hathorn was studying the effects of low oxygen on iron in rats. He was South African and left his country because of the apartheid system there.

Mike Armstrong-James was a neurophysiologist. Ron Spiers was a dental physiologist. Andrew Wade was a veterinary physiologist. Bill Keatinge was working with his Ph.D. student, Jeffrey Graham, on the nerve supply of the arteries of sheep.

As I spent time with my new colleagues, some of them mentioned that Bill Keatinge could be difficult to work with. However, Jeffrey Graham, who had medical degrees, befriended me and could not speak more highly of Bill. Jeff had been a student at Oxford University, where Bill taught until he got the job as Reader in Physiology at the London. Bill was a catch for the department as he had already published a book *Survival in Cold Water* and was known nationally. He was often on the radio after drowning tragedies. I decided to work with Bill and undertake research on aspects of human hypothermia (low body temperature).

I did not really wish to undertake animal research. Most of the other physiologists were undertaking animal research. Andrew Wade, who trained as a vet, was responsible for the animals' welfare. The animals were looked after like gold and never experienced pain. Mice and rats were the majority of the animals used. Cats were anaesthetised and used to demonstrate various aspects of their physiology. They were not allowed to recover from the anaesthetic. Later, these demonstrations were filmed so that not so many cats were used.

There was an ethical committee one had to consult but only if one had doubts as to the ethics of one's experiment. Professor Cross occasionally volunteered for experiments by colleagues who had failed to get that particular work approved by the ethics committee. Some of the experiments he told us about sounded quite dangerous.

Mike Armstrong-James was eventually offered a chair and succeeded Kenneth Cross as the head of department. One was allowed to spend

£10 a day on equipment, and so on. Mike made a computer out of lots of £10 bits of electronics.

Jim Barrowman was replaced by another gastroenterologist, David Wingate. He too became a professor and head of the Wingate Institute of Neurogastroenterology.

In my last year in the department, Dr Hilary Sellick joined me working in my (our) laboratory. She was studying the receptors of lungs of newborn rabbits. Bill had known her in Oxford. She eventually married Andrew Wade, and I was invited to their wedding reception. Her parents were pretty wealthy from the ownership of a dry-cleaning business. When we arrived for the reception, I realised that that building I thought was the house was the 'lodge'. Hilary and Andrew eventually left the department to run their own farm.

There was a mixture of crude and sophisticated scientific instruments, measuring devices, and investigative techniques used in the department. One example was the measurement of radioactivity in the intact rat using a small-animal scintillation counter. Another was atomic absorption spectrophotometry for calcium and magnesium. Some of these instruments were designed and made in-house and were original. Other departments in the medical college and hospital were using a vast array of instruments and measurement techniques. It was possible that a researcher somewhere in the London Hospital complex was using a technique that would be useful to another researcher. About two years after I started working there, I collated a book called *The Catalyst*. It was the third issue.[7] The foreword was written by the professor of medicine, Clifford Wilson, and a quote from this explains the function of this book. 'Different departments—clinical and preclinical—might be using basic scientific techniques which were not only applicable in other fields but might also stimulate new ideas and methods of approach in a wide range of subjects. Ideally this exchange of technical knowledge and discussion of research problems should be by word of mouth at regular

---

[7] Catalyst No. 3. 1972. The London Hospital Medical College. Collated by R. E. G. Sloan.

and frequent inter-departmental meetings. But alas, apart from coffee time (and we should not underestimate the communications value of this ritual) teaching timetables and other commitments make frequent attendance at such meetings almost impossible. All honour therefore to those who devote time and energy to producing "Catalyst" and to the many contributors to the present number.'

The place other than coffee where work was discussed was the Blizard Club. William Blizard was one of the co-founders of the hospital at the end of the eighteenth century. This was where one could have morning coffee, lunch, and afternoon tea if one was a member of staff of the medical college. I occasionally met my friend Brian Colvin there as he was working in the haematology department. I remember having lunch with the professor of neurosurgery, who told us that when a skull had been opened, operating on the brain was like operating on blancmange. I am not sure he should have talked about that sort of thing over a meal. After lunch, I always sat in an armchair and shut my eyes for ten minutes, a habit I kept up until I retired as a GP in 2005.

What was the state of calculating and computing scientific results at that time? We each had a basic calculator in our laboratories. There was a Wang calculator on the floor below us. These were brought out in 1965 and were thought to be somewhat sophisticated as they could deal with logarithms. I once went one floor down where the Wang was kept to divide 1000 by 10! Absent-minded scientist? (Many years before, a professor of anatomy died by falling down a lift shaft not noticing there was no lift after he had opened the outer door.) There was a computer that all of us used extensively. It was the size of a living room and sited about a mile down the Whitechapel Road at Queen Mary's College. We wrote our own computer programmes using the computer language Fortran IV. We typed on a punch card machine a programme instruction and this was produced on a card.

The next instruction produced another card and so on until there was a set of cards with a complete computer programme. The set of cards was kept together with an elastic band and placed in a tray.

Twice a day a man would collect the bundled cards and cycle down the road to the computer. The cards would be returned to you accompanied by a printed sheet with the programme typed out. Quite often, the printed sheet would simply state 'Error on card 52'. It took another day to remedy mistakes. Once one had perfected the computer programme, data cards could be added and perhaps a graph produced. My neighbour Fred Smales became somewhat obsessed with a computer game he had developed and would often stay on late to work on this. I am writing this book using an HP Touchscreen computer with 582 GB of built-in hard disk memory and voice recognition software.

During the first few months of my working in the department, as well as research, I read a lot of basic physiology textbooks to prepare for my teaching commitments.

I was given laboratory space that consisted of a room with working surfaces and shelves, drawers, and so on. Adjoining this was another small room for taking measurements. That room led into another, the atmosphere of which could be heated or cooled down and maintained at a chosen temperature. Bill's last Ph.D. student, Jim Haight, had used the room to study the effects of low blood sugar caused by exercise and ingesting alcohol on temperature regulation in the cold.[8]

The first thing Bill taught me was to realise the importance of the accuracy of any measurements I made. I did not know what the theme of my research would be at this stage, but I knew I would be using thermometers. So how does one know a thermometer used to measure the temperature of my cold room is giving an accurate reading? The thermometer was guaranteed to be accurate by a British standard but that was not good enough for us. I had to calibrate it using a Beckmann thermometer.

---

[8]   J. S. J. Haight and W. R. Keatinge. 1973. *Failure of Thermoregulation in the Cold during Hypoglycaemia Induced by Exercise and Ethanol.* J. Physio. (1973), 229, pp. 87-97.

A Beckmann thermometer measures changes in temperature and has an alterable range of about five degrees. It is accurate to one-hundredth of a degree centigrade. Its range could be set for warm or cool temperatures by altering the level of mercury. Because it can be affected by atmospheric pressure, I used another instrument in the basement of the building to measure this pressure before and after calibration. I heated up a bath of water and kept it at a steady temperature. Into that bath was placed the thermometer I was calibrating and held with a clamp with the Beckmann in another clamp. After about twenty minutes to allow stabilisation, the temperature was noted on the thermometers. The temperature of the bath was then increased by two or three degrees, and after stabilisation, again the temperature of the thermometer in question was noted. The change in temperature in that thermometer was compared with the accurate change in the Beckmann. All this would be repeated at a different temperature of the water bath. I mention this calibration in detail to describe how time consuming some experiments are to ensure accuracy of measurements. This calibration exercise led to my thinking of my first research project.

I started wondering first not only how accurate clinical mercury in glass thermometers were but also how accurate was the measurement of mouth temperatures of patients. Sublingual (under the tongue) temperature measurement was the preferred method for measuring body temperature in patients. I discussed these thoughts with Bill, who was not only my Ph.D. supervisor, but also my co-worker. I became obsessed with this work. We decided that I should study the effects of being in a cool and cold room on sublingual temperature measurements. There was a lot of reading of the literature to be done. Bill got me nominated and elected as a Fellow of the Royal Society of Medicine. This was not an honour but simply allowed me to use one of the largest medical libraries in Europe. To search for papers, the Index Medicus was used. This consisted of a large number of volumes for each year (since the late 1800s) with subjects and authors indexed alphabetically. A new volume was added in a current year every couple of months. The Index Medicus ceased to be published in the printed form in 2004 as it was replaced by computer literature search tools such as Medline. I spent a lot of time in the Royal Society of Medicine library. I was proposing to study the effect of cooling the head on sublingual temperature. The evidence was very strong that oesophageal (the food pipe) temperature accurately reflected deep artery blood temperature. I had to find volunteers who could tolerate the swallowing of an oesophageal probe such that the tip (containing a thermistor for measuring temperature) was sited behind the heart. I found I could swallow this fairly easily. I never did any experiments on anyone that I did not do first on myself. Bill Keatinge volunteered for one of the experiments. After he had swallowed the probe with difficulty, he was in obvious discomfort for the rest of the experiment, his eyes streaming. He never uttered a word of complaint. I advertised for volunteers among medical students and student nurses. Half of them were unable to tolerate swallowing the probe. I met one of the nurses who was unable to swallow the probe several years later. Averil married Stephen Smith, Kath's nephew. Stephen qualified as a doctor at the London. He became a consultant pathologist in Taunton. We have often holidayed with them.

We wondered whether there was an effect of cool saliva on sublingual temperature. We were pretty sure that no one had studied this before. Prof. Ron Spiers, a dental physiologist, got permission for me to use the British Dental Society library. He was very helpful to me. I had to place and fix, by suction, a device that would collect saliva from the duct of the parotid salivary gland on the inner surface of a cheek in the mouth. This was called a Lashley cannula, and we modified it such that temperature measurements could be made of the saliva as it flowed out of the duct. These experiments took months to research and set up. To my horror, I found a reference in the basement of the Royal Society of medicine library in a Russian journal published in 1937.[9] The researcher had put his head in a fridge and measured saliva flow rate, which increased in that cold environment. This was the only reference to saliva for our proposed work. These days with literature searches using electronic databases, it is unlikely that these go as far back so far in time. I know

---

9   Dorodnitsina, A. A. The Influence of Cooling and Heating on the Unconditioned Salivary Reflexes in Man. 1937. Fiz. Zhur. S.S.S.R. 23 (1), pp. 111-16.

that some researchers do not bother to look further back than the time electronic databases cover. I am sure that important information is missed by not looking into old research. Some of the fundamental work on sublingual temperature measurement was published by John Davy in 1845[10] and Carl Wunderlich in 1871.[11]

We showed that there was considerable lowering of the sublingual temperature in cold environments, partly due to an increased flow of cold saliva. We published a paper in the *British Medical Journal*.[12] Publishing our work in peer reviewed journals and demonstrating experiments to the Physiological Society was a wise move of Bill. It meant that the Ph.D. thesis of mine had, in large part, already been accepted by experts and that I was almost bound to attain the qualification.

Bill and I met weekly to discuss ideas and make plans. We also met over coffee. He was doing work with his Ph.D. student, Jeff Graham, on the smooth muscle of sheep's arteries. Every morning Jeff would arrive with a bit of sheep's artery that was fresh from the slaughterhouse. I never really understood what they were looking at, but it was pretty high-powered stuff. Bill occasionally sent his work for comments to Andrew Huxley, the Nobel Prize winner who taught me at University College. Bill taught me never to be too proud to ask advice. Indeed, we got advice from a professor of statistics on how to deal with some of our results.

This work on sublingual temperatures led us to develop a thermometer that measured temperature from a probe inserted into the ear canal (the aural or auditory canal). However, we showed that the aural canal was also subject to local cooling. We therefore insulated the ear with a heat pad that was maintained at the same temperature as the probe. I

---

[10] John Davy. 1845. *On the Temperature of Man.* Phil. Trans. R. Soc. Lond. 135, pp. 319-33.

[11] Wunderlich, C. A. and Seguin, E. 1871. *Medical Thermometry and Human Temperature.* New York: William Wood and Co.

[12] Sloan, R. E. G. and Keatinge, W. R. 1975. *Depression of Sublingual Temperature by Cold Saliva.* B. M. J. Mar 75; 1 (5960), pp. 718-20.

could not have done this work without the fantastic help of the senior electronics technician, Tony Barnett. He was a great character with a unique sense of humour. He told me he kept a 'black book' with notes about any academic who upset him and how he could delay their projects. It was a good job that we got on very well. Tony would not allow any of the physiologists to change a light bulb. He maintained that academic physiologists were not trained to change light bulbs. Once he ordered an electronic component from the USA and labelled the request as 'extremely urgent—for medical use.' It was flown over on Concord.

The prototype thermometer we used in experiments in my cold room was about five feet tall, one foot deep, and three feet wide. It was really a set of shelves on which measuring and recording instruments could be placed and supplied with electricity. This could be wheeled from my lab to the ante-room next to the temperature-controlled room where the volunteer was. Testing the 'thermometer' involved using the oesophageal temperature as a reference. I will not go into the details of these experiments, which took about a year to complete. However, the method of lowering the deep body temperature was to have the volunteer in swimming costume with the legs immersed in cold water. The rest of the body was in warmish air. The feet moved backwards and forwards on a pedal such that the cooler blood in the calves was pumped up. At the same time, heat was lost from the rest of the body to the warmer room as a result of its blood vessels widening in response to the heat.

When we were sure that this prototype thermometer was reliable, I approached a company, Muirhead Ltd, that had an excellent reputation for manufacturing accurate scientific instruments. It was the start of a fascinating experience working with industry and developing an instrument that would be sold on the open market. My initial contacts were Messrs Spray and Sieber and their director was Ron Griffin. The machine that was developed was portable and called the zero gradient aural thermometer (ZGAT).

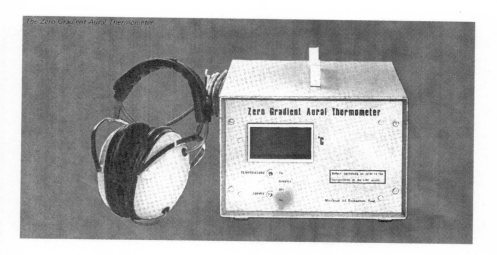

The zero-gradient aural thermometer.

Bill decided that I should demonstrate the device at the Physiological Society. This resulted in my being a nervous wreck for weeks, but it is another way of publishing the work. We had to take the tank and the portable device up to Oxford. Adrian Jacobs, Bill's technician, volunteered to be the experimental subject. We took all the equipment up in Bill's estate car. Bill's driving left a lot to be desired as he had the habit of outlining graphs, and so on, with his finger on the inside of the windscreen while travelling at speed. We set the experiment up in the morning, and Adrian had his legs in the tank for about two hours while eminent physiologists wondered in and out of the room and stopped to ask questions if they wished. To my horror, I saw Prof. Andrew Huxley, the Nobel Prize winner, approaching. I tried to hide. He obviously did not recognise me as one of his former students and actually was charming. His question was easy to answer. A summary of the demonstration was published in the *Journal of Physiology* but only after members of the Physiological Society had voted it through.[13]

---

13   W. R. Keatinge and R. E. G. Sloan. 1973. *Measurement of Deep Body Temperature from External Auditory Canal with Servo-Controlled Heating around Ear*. Proceedings of the Physiological Society, 13-14 July. Journal of Physiology, 234, pp. 8-9.

The ZGAT was sold all over the world including one to NASA. It was spotted in a report on the BBC's scientific programme, 'Tomorrow's World'. It was the first invention to earn royalties for the London Hospital. The demonstration to the Physiological Society in Oxford was in 1973. The latest reference in the literature for its use to measure deep body temperature is 1999. It had a good run until superseded by tympanic membrane thermometers, used today by almost all clinicians. I seriously question whether these have been researched rigorously.

I worked in the physiology department for about three years, and my next job was as a partner in a general practice in Cheltenham. Shortly after starting work in that town, I was approached by Ron Griffin (director at Muirhead Ltd) to join him at an Anglo-Italian medical congress in Florence. The meeting was for business people rather than scientists and was organised by diplomats. It was February 1974. The firm paid my expenses and that of the practice to employ a locum for my absence for about two weeks. We were to have a stand to show off and sell the ZGAT. Ron had significant business connections with Italy and spoke Italian. He always drove to Italy. We started very early. To my horror, he put on a tape of Nazi marching tunes as we set off. I wondered what on earth he was like. I did not really know Ron at all so was somewhat anxious about the whole trip. In my mind, businessmen abroad spent their evenings in strip clubs and brothels. He drove at 50 miles per hour, and we drove about 500 miles the first day. We did not stop more than a few minutes for lunch or to go to the lavatory. We arrived at our overnight stop at Geneva—the Hotel Intercontinental. This was and still is a luxury hotel. We ate in a superb restaurant on the top floor with magnificent views. We were departing early the next day so I ordered a slap-up breakfast in my room as I knew we would not be having much lunch. When I met Ron in the lobby, he asked me what I had for breakfast. I told him and he said he had had a glass of water. This was because he had found out how much the bill for the hotel was before he went to sleep. It was so expensive that we did not have lunch for the rest of our time in Italy. The cost of a basic room in that hotel at the time of writing is about £390 a night excluding breakfast. We arrived in Florence in the evening. We stayed at the Grand Hotel

Minerva in the Piazza di Santa Maria Novella. It was a four-star hotel close to where the congress was being held. The next morning, we set off to set up our stand and Ron carried the ZGAT. The handle was such that it was uncomfortable and Ron became seriously angry and telephoned Muirhead to order the handles to be changed.

We set up our stand and sat there each of the ten days of the congress. We got to know one another very well. I was quite wrong about what businessmen do in the evening. The ones I met first phoned their wives and then went out for a nice meal. We went to the same restaurant most nights but twice we treated ourselves to a meal at Ristorante Otello, which was founded in 1934 and is still there at the time of writing.

A UK General Election took place while we were there. On the day of the election, the diplomats who had been swanning about the congress disappeared into thin air. We sat up late into the night in the hotel foyer (we could get radio reception nowhere else in the hotel) listening to the results on a small radio. We asked the night porter to turn the florescent lights off so we could get better reception. It was a very exciting election that resulted in Harold Wilson forming a minority government in a hung parliament. At one point when we had no radio reception, I telephoned the British Embassy in Rome for the latest. The man who answered told me that he had no idea and was writing a letter. It was 2 a.m.

The ZGAT hit the local press but we made no sales. It would have been a totally boring experience but that Ron and I had plenty to talk about to one another. On the last day, the stand was approached by an Italian ear, nose, and throat specialist wearing his jacket in Italian style—over his shoulders. He was followed a few paces behind by his junior colleagues. He asked Ron 'Canna you putta de prob uppa de nose?' Ron replied, 'You can stick it up your arse, if you want.' We packed up the stand and prepared to go home.

In the early evening of the last night, we were invited to a reception on the top floor of the beautiful Palazzo Vecchio in the Piazza della Signoria.

I had to be back at work and Ron said I could travel home by any means I chose. I chose to reserve a first-class seat on a train from Florence to Calais. I learnt the hard way that Italians have no respect for reserved seats, and I stood up for the first three hours. Then the heating failed, and I slept under a Frenchman's overcoat. When I arrived in Calais, the boat I was due to board had set off and was about five metres from the keyside. At least I had a comfortable first-class train journey from Dover to London.

I loved Florence so much that Felicity, my first wife, and I returned in the summer and stayed in the same hotel. The barman remembered me and my favourite drink—a dry martini cocktail.

Bill felt I had not yet enough material for a Ph.D. I had been to see someone who was organising some children to swim the English Channel. Hardly anything was known about the effects of children swimming in cold water, and Bill felt that the channel swim could be dangerous. We warned the organiser and decided to have no further involvement. We designed a huge experiment that took at least six months to prepare, a morning to perform and six months to analyse. The effects of swimming in an indoor pool in coolish water (20.3 °C) were studied in sixteen girls and twelve boys aged eight to nineteen. We used Wandsworth swimming pool that had cooled down somewhat after being closed for Easter. They swam for up to forty minutes, and anyone appearing unduly cold got out early. Measurements had to be made of temperatures, height, weight, skinfold thickness, and metabolic rate (in some). Swim speeds were measured. The number of observers taking all these measurements was many. It included Kenneth Cross, head of department and his wife, my wife, technicians including the chief, Geoff Watling. The experiment was funded in part by the Royal Naval Personnel Research Committee. One of the observers was Surgeon Lt Cdr Frank Golden, who was a physiologist and had worked with Bill in the past.

What did we find out? Subcutaneous fat was the main factor related to cooling rates, but the surface area/mass ratio also played a part. One thin boy's temperature dropped to 34.4 °C and one fat girl's rose to 37.7 °C. The lower temperatures were accompanied by considerable shivering. We have all seen thin boys coming out of the cold sea shivering violently with their teeth clattering. Fat thickness was less and falls in temperature were greater in young than older swimmers and in boys than girls.

I gave a ten-minute presentation of these results at the Physiological Society held in Aberdeen in July 1972.[14] I stayed a night at Bill's house before we travelled to Scotland the next day. He had just arrived back from Canada and had brought a whole salmon. The salmon was in a cool bag, and Bill had this with him the whole of the flight. His daughter announced she did not like Salmon and Bill went to bed exasperated and with jet lag. I smoked cigarettes at that time and was dreading having to abstain while staying at Bill's house. However, to my delight, Bill's then wife Annette also smoked and had put an ashtray for me on my bedside table. We flew up to Aberdeen the next day and spent the next night in student accommodation. I found the presentation experience nerve-racking as questions could be asked by very eminent scientists. Then a vote is taken as to whether the work can be published. When I returned to London, I discovered that my car had been stolen from the car park at Heathrow Airport. (While a student and working in London, I had every car I owned stolen. I got them all back except for the one after the Aberdeen trip. It was used in a robbery; I learnt much later.)

It is traditional that authors of papers appear in alphabetical order. I light-heartedly accused Bill of, generally, only ever working with people with surnames later in the alphabet than his. We published our results in a full paper in the *Journal of Applied Physiology* written by Sloan and Keatinge.[15] Bill was a generous gentleman, and I never heard him utter a rude word. That paper has been cited many times since publication and

---

[14] W. R. Keatinge and R. E. G. Sloan. 1972. *Effect of Swimming in Cold Water on Body Temperatures of Children.* Proceedings of the Physiological Society. *Journal of Physiology*, 226, pp. 55-6.

[15] R. E. G. Sloan and W. R. Keatinge. 1973. *Cooling Rates of Young People Swimming in Cold Water. J. Appl. Physiol.* 35 (3), pp. 371-5

as recently as 2010 has been described as seminal by Prof. Mike Tipton, a physiologist at the University of Portsmouth.

At the same time as undertaking research, I had a significant teaching commitment—lectures, tutorials, and running practical classes.

Readers might have gathered by now that I tend to get significantly anxious about things. I was a nervous wreck thinking about undertaking my first lecture to around 100 medical students. I remembered how we behaved in lectures as students: not very politely. I spent weeks writing out the first lecture and even had in parentheses on several occasions 'pause for laughter'. I had to do a lot of reading around my subject as lots had changed since I last studied physiology at University College. I struggled to understand some of it and prayed I would not be asked to explain those areas. Slides were made for me to show in a lecture. There was a blackboard and chalk. There were certainly none of the audio—visual aids available today. This detailed preparation in the first year took up significant research time. However, unless new topics were given to me in subsequent years, the lectures could be repeated after updating them. Eventually, I felt more confident and could ad-lib some humour and give real-life examples to illustrate. I tried to model myself on the lecturers who had taught me and whom I regarded as excellent. I lectured on the physiology of the kidney, endocrines (hormones), and the heart. I knew that if one learnt how the body works under normal conditions, that greatly helped understanding the effect of diseases on the body.

Each term I looked after a different tutorial group of about twelve students. There were not enough teaching staff to undertake one-to-one tutorials. Occasionally, I would undertake a one-to-one tutorial for a student in difficulty. The London Hospital Medical College had a policy of taking mature students (who had, for example, been in the armed forces or a job) and these greatly enhanced the groups. You will see in a later chapter that I really learnt about running a group only when I was becoming a teacher in general practice. The tutorials were held weekly and essays were set. I caught one student out for copying (plagiarism).

At some point in his essay, he had written 'see page 56'. I went through every text book I could until I found the page. I realised that honesty was the best policy, and if I did not know anything, I promised to find out. Mutual respect between teacher and student was a great thing that I learnt from both J. Z. Young and Bill.

There were practical classes, and we physiology teachers facilitated these. There was an explanation as to what was to be done was followed by my being available for queries and walking among the students. A senior technician was also at hand. These classes lasted half and sometimes the whole day. I was in charge of the class on the kidney. This involved the students drinking a significant amount of water and then measuring the urine output and other aspects of the urine for a number of hours after. The class was divided into two. One half was given an injection of antidiuretic hormone (ADH) also known as vasopressin. This hormone was part of the control mechanism regulating how much urine was passed. Its effect is to reduce urine output. The reason it was also called vasopressin is because it causes small arteries to constrict and a rise in blood pressure. The practical class usually ran smoothly, but one year I had to admit a student to the hospital medical unit. He had had an injection of ADH. He developed a significant fever. This could simply have been a flu-like illness, but as a temperature man, I wanted to investigate this further. I decided to do an experiment on myself. I sat in my temperature-controlled room (in a coolish environment) for thirty minutes and took oesophageal temperature readings. I then injected myself with ADH. Indeed, my temperature rose significantly. Narrowing of the blood vessels in the skin prevents heat loss. The only other time there was a medical problem with a student was with one of my research volunteers. He developed an irregular heartbeat as I was cooling him down. I got Bill to examine him. It was nothing serious, but we abandoned the experiment on him. The student I admitted with a fever made a full recovery and nothing serious was discovered.

Towards the end of my third year working with Bill, we were planning further research. I had now enough material to write up my Ph.D. He had forgotten that I told him at the start of my time with him that I intended to be a GP. I had been approached by my good friend Robin Harrod, who was a GP in Cheltenham. There was a partnership vacancy, and it had been offered to me. Bill was somewhat shocked but hardly showed it as he was always the perfect gentleman. I started writing up the thesis in that third year and completed it while working as a partner in Cheltenham. In those days, generally, GPs worked in the morning and had a break until the evening surgery starting at 4 p.m. I wrote the thesis in the early afternoons. I paid a local firm to make high-quality graphs and tables and another company to make four hard-bound copies. Bill gave me feedback on my writing as I was going along. When printed, the Ph.D. thesis was submitted to the University of London.

The last stage of a Ph.D. is the viva. There were two examiners, my supervisor Bill and an external examiner. Bill approached Prof. W. I. Cranston, MD, FRCP. He was the professor of medicine at St Thomas's Hospital and an expert on body temperature regulation. We had quoted his work on ear temperatures in our papers. I knew that the viva could last up to three hours. The outcome was either a pass, a fail, or a request to resubmit the thesis. The Ph.D. viva could not be repeated. One could be asked to undertake a five-hour practical examination. I travelled to London from Cheltenham for the viva and was so nervous that Bill told me to go for a walk in the Whitechapel Road. All went well and Professor Cranston was charming. The viva lasted about ninety minutes. Bill dug me out of the occasional hole. The night before the viva I had noticed an error in one of the graphs and had printed a corrected version. I told Professor Cranston this at the end of the viva and he asked me to get some glue so we could stick it over the erroneous graph. We stuck it in, and when I shook hands with him to say goodbye, I had some glue on the palm of my right hand. We nearly stuck together. We laughed.

I had been to two University of London degree ceremonies, one for the B.Sc. and the second for the MB, BS. These are held in the Albert Hall. My mother and her cousin Yella Giles were the two guests I was allowed for these. The chancellor of the university at that time was

Queen Elizabeth, the Queen Mother. However, on each occasion, the vice chancellor awarded the degrees.

The higher degree ceremony was a different ball game. It was held in the Senate House of the University of London. My mother and my first wife, Felicity, were my guests. There was string quartet playing for the reception. We were served delicate sandwiches and a drink before the ceremony. I had hired the rather magnificent robe.

The robe of a doctor of science was even more ornate. Again the vice chancellor presented. This was the first of the three career highlights of my career. The other two were being nominated as a Fellow of the Royal College of General Practitioners and being awarded an MBE.

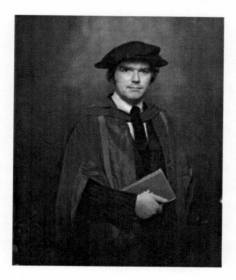

The London University Ph.D. robe.

Next stop, general practice.

CHAPTER 7

GENERAL PRACTICE IN CHELTENHAM AND LONDON

My good friend and best man at my first wedding, Robin Harrod, had been a partner in a practice in Cheltenham for three years or so. Felicity had qualified and had nearly finished her pre-registration house jobs. It was 1973. Robin told me that there was a vacancy in his practice in Cheltenham. He asked me to consider the job. It was perfect timing. I had always wanted to be a GP, and I had started to write my Ph.D. thesis. I went to Cheltenham and had an informal meeting with the partners who offered me the job. I was part of what was known as the 'gold rush'. The government had announced that in order to practise as a GP, one had to undertake a further three years of vocational training. This would involve a year of attachments to training general practices as well as hospital jobs. I certainly did not want to spend another period training. I had already spent ten years getting to this point. I therefore 'rushed' into becoming a GP.

Further experience in obstetrics was required before a GP was allowed on the obstetric list. This enabled a GP to be paid for looking after pregnant women, deliveries, and post-natal patients. There were two ways of being included on the obstetric list. The first was to undertake a six-month senior house officer post in obstetrics. This was the route most potential GPs took. The other was to be attached to an obstetric unit for six months or so. I mentioned that the academic staff in the physiology department could come and go as they pleased. I arranged with a consultant obstetrician in Barnet General Hospital to undertake such an attachment. This involved my attending antenatal outpatient clinics once a week and living in the hospital one night a week. I had to deliver twenty babies and watch some abnormal deliveries. Towards the end, when the senior house officer took a week's holiday, I did her locum. This attachment was great experience, and I think I have delivered more babies (about forty) than most GP colleagues. I was admitted to the obstetric list. During that locum job, it hit home that I had not dealt with a patient for three years. I had been in a laboratory.

I spent the weeks before starting at the Leckhampton Road Surgery swotting up medicine again. I had forgotten how to treat a sore throat or to issue a certificate of unfitness to work. Dai James, the retiring partner, was only in his early forties when he decided to run a dog kennel business. He wrote me a postcard with what he felt was all one needed to know to practise as a GP. In the top left-hand corner was an area labelled 'Skins'. He wrote, 'anything that itches, betnovate. Scabies, benzyl benzoate application'.

The Leckhampton Road Surgery was an old building and may have been listed. An incoming partner was expected to buy a share from the outgoing partner. The cost to me of becoming a quarter owner of the surgery was about £5,000. My generous mother gave me that as a present. The central heating was run by a solid fuel boiler. The partner who was on duty for the weekend had the job of 'clinking' the boiler on Saturday and Sunday. This was shaking the coke ashes to the bottom of the fire by means of a handle on the side of the boiler. There were four partners—Robin Harrod, Dick Anthony, the senior partner Tony Mules, and I. The practice had about 10,000 patients mainly in Cheltenham but also some in rural places such as the village of Birdlip. There was very rarely a visit request to Birdlip as the villagers were hardened country folk. We each had a consulting room and a separate examination room. My consulting room was on the ground floor (as was Robin's). It was next to reception, and I could overhear what was being said in there.

One of the receptionists, Joan Preston, also from Yorkshire, had the habit of always asking, 'Is it urgent?' I occasionally told patients how to get around this. 'If you want to speak to a doctor, tell the receptionist you are his second cousin. 'If you want an appointment or a visit, mention blood.' My room also had a door that opened to the street. I mainly used this to let out patients who had been tearful in the consultation. Robin and I maintained that we saw all the knee and hip arthritis cases as they had difficulty getting up the stairs to the other partners. The practice was one of the first in the UK to employ a practice nurse, Mary Mayo. She was a great character, and we both had the honour of being asked to be godparents to Robin and Christine Harrod's second child Samantha. Dai James was also her godfather. Occasionally, on a Friday evening after surgery, the four partners would meet with her in Tony's room and get stuck into several gin and tonics. As the early evening progressed, Mary would phone each of our wives to explain that we were running late and would be home soon. Once, we got pretty drunk, and some of us got into serious trouble when we eventually arrived back home. I was one of them. It really was very bad behaviour.

The staff we employed were hard working, loyal, and some of them had worked there for many years. I was asked to be the partner responsible for staff management. This was no easy job as I was so inexperienced. The long-standing secretary, Joyce Peeters, left after one of my bad decisions. So did the practice manager, Margaret Norman. Joyce got a job with another general practice, but I persuaded her to return to us, which was a great relief as she was excellent. Margaret retired permanently.

There was the perennial problem that appointments were difficult to get and the system seemed not to cope. Robin and I talked at length about different models of appointment systems. We heard of one surgery that doubled the number of appointments. This made no difference whatsoever. After a two-hour morning surgery, there would be 'extras' to see, which we shared out. We then all met in Tony's room for coffee and to share the visits. The number of these varied, and if there were not very many, coffee time could be a protracted affair. We signed the repeat prescriptions during the coffee break and messages were dealt with. The repeat prescriptions were written out by hand by a member of the administrative staff, and we checked and signed them. There was another safety check made by the pharmacist.

Patients collected their prescriptions from the surgery and could take them to the pharmacy of their choice. GPs have a close relationship with their local pharmacy. Ours was Leckhampton Pharmacy owned by Tom Critchley. It was situated near our surgery and most of our patients used it. Each partner had a personal account at his chemist shop. Anything bought on our accounts was allowed against tax as these were put on to the practice accounts. We certainly took liberties with what we bought there. Tom was a widower and was always invited to practise Christmas parties. After my marriage broke down, I went out with him a couple of times for dinner at his favourite place, the Moorend Park Hotel.

An appointment was seven and a half minutes and double appointments could be made for procedures such as gynaecological examinations or minor surgery. It was easy to fill one's appointments up by telling the patient to come and see you again to check on something. If an appointment with a GP was especially difficult to obtain, the patient might think, 'Wow, that doctor must be brilliant because everybody wants to see him. He's always full up'. I used to tease Robin that he filled his appointments up with follow-up patients. The truth was, of course, that Robin was an excellent GP.

Unless you were the duty doctor on call for emergencies, the afternoon was free until the evening surgery, which was from 4 to 6 p.m. I wrote my Ph.D. up in the afternoons. My next door neighbour, consultant neurologist David Stevens, envied this time I had as he worked really hard from morning to when he got home, often late in the evening.

We worked alternate Saturday mornings with one partner being the duty doctor until 6 p.m. Saturday morning was spent undertaking private medical examinations often for insurance companies. I will explain how GPs were paid and about their contract with the National Health Service later. Another partner took over on Saturday evening and continued to work over the weekend until surgery opened on Monday morning. This involved about thirteen weekends a year. It was my job to sort out the duty rota from a set of eighteen cards each with a different set of circumstances for holidays, and so on. I thought a computer might be able to sort this better, and I took the cards to a software firm. I was told it was far too complicated.

We continued to go to social events while on duty and were not very good at refraining from alcohol when on call. I very rarely accepted an alcoholic drink from a patient, but on one Christmas day when I was on call, I made an exception. I had had a couple of sherries and a mince pie in a house. On leaving, I opened the door and called goodbye and shut the door behind me to find I had shut myself in a cupboard.

Felicity and I bought a three-storey town house in The Park, Cheltenham. Soon after moving in, I met my neighbour, David. He asked me what my job was and was somewhat taken aback when I told him. He had just been appointed as a consultant neurologist. I think he would have preferred to not have a doctor living next door. I was disturbed when we disclosed our salaries to one another that David was paid slightly less than me despite his training for nearly a decade more than me. My salary at that time was just over £5,000 per annum. David and Ute Stevens were great neighbours. However, I seriously upset David on one occasion. We were at a dinner party, and I argued that a coal miner was more valuable to society than a consultant neurologist. David did not speak to me for a long time. A few years later, both Robin and Christine and David and Ute moved house and ended up next-door neighbours. I learnt a lot from David about neurology, and at one time he was considering employing me as a clinical assistant undertaking nerve conduction studies. This never came off. Another job offer from a consultant surgeon also never came off. He enquired whether I was any good with my hands. I asked what he meant. He said, 'Can you change the fuse of an electric plug?' When I told him I could, he offered me a clinical assistantship with him doing gastroscopies (looking into and examining the inside of the stomach). I declined as I was unhappy with anything surgical.

GPs at that time were self-employed with a contract to work for the National Health Service. The contract required a practice to provide emergency cover for their patients twenty-four hours a day, 365 days a year. How one organised surgeries and cover was entirely up to the practice, which was really a small business. GPs could undertake other jobs in addition to their NHS work, such as working at the hospital, insurance company medicals, and private patients. Robin did some occupational health work for a group of factories. Tony was the medical adviser for the Cheltenham branch of Marks and Spencer.

The administration of GPs, pharmacists, and opticians was undertaken by a relatively small number of people working for the Family Practitioner Committee (FPC). This was the local administrative body of the NHS. How a GP was paid was set out in a loose-leafed booklet called 'The Red Book'. It outlined the terms and conditions of service for a GP or group of GPs as well as the payments and how to claim. There were many different forms to complete and send in, some having to be signed by the patient. There was a basic salary, payment for being on the obstetric list, and seniority payments (after working as a GP for a number of specified years). There were then additional items of service payments. Here are some examples of item of service claims that could be submitted: giving contraceptive advice; undertaking a smear; looking after a patient in a rural area; giving advice to a temporary resident; visiting a patient in a lighthouse; visiting a patient where one had to walk to get to the house. Each one of these items had a separate claim form to complete.

We had private patients. We did not want anyone to be financially compromised by becoming a private patient of a GP. Our private patients were very wealthy, and we charged a significant amount for our time. The time spent on private patients did not encroach on NHS work. To become a private patient, he or she had to write to the FPC and withdraw from NHS general practice care. This meant the cost of medicines written on private prescriptions had to be paid in full. This could be very expensive. My private patients included a junior member of the Saudi royal family and his staff. It was fascinating for me to see such wealth and experience of the medical problems that were presented to me by them. Once I was asked to travel from Cheltenham to London to see a relation of theirs who had a sore throat. At the time of writing, I am wearing the valuable Omega watch that was given to me by them. Any money paid to us by private patients went into the partnership pot.

Most of the consultants working in Cheltenham and nearby Gloucester had flourishing private practices. There was a private hospital (The Nuffield) in Cheltenham. One consultant general surgeon lived in the country on his farm. He threw an annual party. It was rumoured that GPs were invited only if they had supplied him with £1,000 of private work in the past year. I was never invited. One winter, in heavy snow, I was called out to a man with a strangulated inguinal hernia. This is a surgical emergency. The patient asked to be admitted privately and Steve Haynes was the duty consultant surgeon. Steve was housebound because of the snow. He asked me to look after the patient overnight. He told me to give the patient an injection of morphine and prop the foot of the bed up. Steve came into the hospital the next morning. Everything turned out well. The only other time I was in charge of a private patient in the Nuffield was one of mine who had had a heart attack and was in the intensive care unit in Cheltenham General Hospital. He asked me to transfer him to the private Nuffield hospital so he could smoke his cigarettes. This I did. The consultants did not like my using one of 'their' beds. On occasions on Saturday morning, we could assist a consultant in the operating theatre. I only did this once as I disliked anything to do with surgery. The operation was on a patient I had referred. It was an interesting experience being able to talk about the operation with the patient later. I was paid for that work.

The bulk of the family planning work was undertaken by Robin and me. The department of health introduced an item of service payment for each patient given contraceptive advice. This mainly involved prescribing the contraceptive pill. There were higher payments for inserting a coil or cap. Robin trained so he could fit coils, and I learnt how to insert caps. Very few women wanted caps so I eventually became deskilled. There were a significant number requesting coils and Robin fitted a lot. After a coil has been inserted, the patient is advised to lie down for five minutes. Robin was somewhat stressed after he had inserted his first coil, and he too felt like lying down for five minutes. These days most of the family planning work is undertaken by nurses and women GPs.

After a couple of years, Robin and I thought we should have another partner and that this should be a woman. We had to persuade Tony, who had indicated in the past that he was not at all keen on working with a woman. 'They have period pains and babies!' The partners' meeting for this venture was held in my house. Robin and I told Tony that as the senior partner he ought to chair the meeting. He had never done that sort of thing. We were trying to have a more business-like approach to decision making. After all, we were small business. We had prominently displayed a couple of articles on the benefits of having a woman GP so that Tony could not avoid seeing them. When Tony arrived, I opened the front door and he was holding a clipboard with some blank sheets of paper. I think he felt that was how a chairman of a meeting should look. All went well, and we decided to advertise for another partner. We had very few applicants and we chose Dr Kate Curtis, who had last worked as a GP in Manchester. She certainly could talk. The partnership with her did not work out. We reread her application after she left and found that her main referee had stated, 'she is a brilliant conversationalist'. That was one way of putting it. She was popular with the patients, likeable, and sociable, and it was a shame the partnership had to be dissolved.

All the GPs in Cheltenham used a branch surgery in a housing estate called Hesters Way. I was asked to be the secretary of that group of doctors and my main objective was to keep the rent low. The rent was paid to the FPC. I was advised that if we were informed of a rent increase, I should write back and complain about something such as a radiator not working properly. This would delay the rent increase for a number of months at which point I complained about something else.

At one point, I arranged an evening meeting for the GPs with the chief administrator of the FPC to thrash out the rent issue. The meeting ended in tragedy. The chief administrator collapsed and died despite attempts to resuscitate him. The local newspaper, the Gloucestershire Echo, reported, 'He died amongst his friends'.

One time the senior partner Tony was ill, and I went up to Hesters Way to do his surgery. I had the arrogance of youth and did not realise how popular Tony was. The patients all went home as they really loved him. Did they think I was useless or too young to understand? Tony was a really good GP to them. Tony had been in the Burma campaign in the Second World War and had marched through the jungle with a malaria fever. He never came to terms with patients phoning in for a visit for a mild feverish illness.

I continued an interest in research as a GP. The Royal College of General Practitioners had developed a card index system, which was used to develop an age—sex register. There were pink cards for females and blue for males. The cards were filed in date of birth order with males and females separately. One could then add a colour tag at the top of the card to indicate, for example, a patient with diabetes. If the cards were kept in open files, one could observe the age—sex distribution of a disease and compare this with published information. One might have discovered we were not diagnosing as many diabetics as we should and that we should be measuring more sugar levels of patients. The practice would have to buy 10,000 cards and employ someone to set it up. The cost would be about £400. My idea was turned down flat by the senior partners on cost grounds. I put my thinking cap on and did a small pilot. I discovered that there were patients attending the surgery that were not registered as patients. We were not being paid at all for them despite having their medical records. I worked out that if we set up an age—sex register, it would not only cover the cost of that but also make a profit. The partners' eyes lit up when I told them, and I was allowed to go ahead. The age—sex register was put together by two medical students and the practice administrative staff. This ensured that we had an accurate record of our patients. The process revealed that ninety-five patients were attending the surgery that were not registered as patients. We were not being paid for seeing them. Registering them easily paid for the age—sex register. This work was published as a research paper in the *Journal of the Royal College of General Practitioners*.[16]

The age—sex register was the start of a larger piece of research for which I obtained funding. One could apply for a locally organised research grant. At that time, these grants were very rarely requested by GPs. The study I embarked on involved identifying the children who had had an epileptic fit associated with a fever and then interviewing their mothers about their experiences with this. The grant I received covered some administration work by our practice manager, Margaret Norman, as well as money equivalent to my being a hospital clinical assistant. That money was paid into the practice and enabled me to work one afternoon a week for over a year on this research. There was also funding for a research assistant. I advertised, and there were about 400 replies including one from an ex-butler and another from a woman with a degree in ballistic science. I took on Mrs Dawn Adams, who had a nursing background and was married to a fellow Cheltenham GP, Jamie. We worked well together. The interviews with mothers revealed amazing stories. One mother ran out of her house with her fitting child and stopped a lorry that was driven at speed to the hospital. Another was reassured so much by the GP about the first fit that she never bothered the doctor any more and her child had been fitting regularly for a number of years. I regret never having written up this work.

Robin became a trainer of GPs and his first trainee was Richard Baker. Richard Baker OBE, MD, FRCGP is, at the time of writing, a professor of quality in health care at the University of Leicester. He once told me that my interest in research started him in his research career, but I have my doubts. He took over my partnership after I left.

---

[16] Sloan, R. E. G., Norman, M. and Adams, D. 1977. *The Cost and Advantages of Establishing an Age-Sex Register.* J. Roy. Col. Gen. Pract. 27, (182): 522-3.

The NHS work was greatly different from that which I undertook in the first few years of this century before I retired in 2005. Strokes and uncomplicated heart attacks were looked after at home. There were lots of visit requests, and we revisited regularly. There were emergency visits to acute asthma and an injection was usually required as part of the treatment. There were emergency visits to diabetic comas and significantly more limbs were amputated in diabetic patients. Emergency psychiatry visits were a worry because of the fear of violence. I often left my car keys in the ignition and the car doors unlocked when visiting certain psychiatric cases. A psychiatric patient once sprayed me all over with perfume using an atomiser. I visited another patient with a consultant and the trainee GP. That patient told us was receiving instructions from the television. As we were leaving, he said, 'Something is going to happen to each of you to do with your cars within the next twenty-four hours'. I had a minor accident and the trainee had something stolen from his car. This was eerie. I telephoned the psychiatrist, and to my relief nothing had happened to him or his car. It was all just a coincidence.

Admitting patients to hospital sometimes was difficult. Psychiatric patients were required to be sectioned (a legal process that enforced an admission to hospital) for three days. The psychiatric unit would not accept voluntary admissions. This was unethical, and we should have fought against it.

On one occasion, Robin wanted to admit a patient to the geriatric hospital. They refused and said that the admission should be under the consultant psycho-geriatrician. The latter consultant refused admission and told Robin to go back to the consultant geriatrician. It became a stalemate situation. Robin decided to report these two consultants to the department of geriatrics at Bristol. The professor of geriatrics came out and summoned the Cheltenham consultants to a meeting having assessed the patient who by this time had to be strapped into a chair at mealtimes. The professor made his decision and it was sorted out. However, for quite a while, Robin had trouble getting his patients into the geriatric hospital. Consultants were not used to being disagreed with. However, GPs are independent self-employed contractors whose patients come first.

Our marriage did not work out, and Felicity and I divorced. I decided to leave Cheltenham and become a physiologist again in the London Hospital. This turned out to be a mistake, and I left my job as a lecturer in physiology after only one week. (This episode I have omitted from my CV!) Bill Keatinge, my Ph.D. supervisor, was, as usual, a true gentleman when I did that. He had gone to a lot of trouble to get me that job. We remained friends until his untimely death in 2008.

I re-met my now wife Kathleen (I mentioned in Chapter 2 that we went out when we were students). We married in 1978 and have been happily married ever since.

We moved into a flat in Roehampton, London, owned by a school friend of my mother. She was Mourussia Borme-Reed, the solicitor who dealt with my divorce. Round the corner was the surgery and house of the Drs. Tintner, the close friends of my parents. They had offered me a job as an assistant with a view to becoming a partner. The patients were, like in Cheltenham, a great mix of the socially deprived and middle class. There was a thriving private practice, and the patients included a couple of nationally famous actors. The only other members of staff were a couple of women who covered reception.

The practice had no appointments system, and I worked in a small consulting room situated between the Tintners' rooms. The surgery was on the ground floor of the house, and the Tintners lived on the first floor. To call a patient, I had to open the door to the waiting room and say 'next patient, please'. To my horror, on many occasions, no one would get up as they wished to see the Tintners. They were very popular. I got the patients in the waiting room to laugh by saying, 'Honestly. I really am a doctor. I will show you my certificates, if you want'. That usually resulted in someone taking pity on me. Because I was the new boy, I had to do all the menial tasks such as ear syringing and injections. Gerda (Beba) took all the phone calls out of hours and sometimes even when she was doing a surgery. She took all the phone calls in the evening and during the night and would then phone me in the flat to give me a visit. There was another partner, Dr Hughes, who called Beba 'mission control'. One excellent practice of Beba was to phone patients up and ask how they were getting on. She maintained that this not only was a nice thing to do but also saved work.

Beba had been in a group of GPs who had undertaken some research with a very famous psychiatrist, Michael Balint. He was at University College Hospital and led this group. The doctors looked at themselves and their psychological and psychiatric make-up. He maintained that by doing this, a GP understands himself or herself better and can deal with patients better. There is today a Balint Society that facilitates meetings every year. His book, *The Doctor, His Patient and the Illness* is a classic.[17] On the Balint Society Web pages, someone has written 'Sounds a bit sexist. What about the doctor and her Patient?' Gerda Tintner was in Balint's original group and was the only woman GP. She is mentioned in the book, which tries to anonymise the GPs. Henry Tintner was really angry when the book was published as one can identify Beba as Balint refers to her as 'she' or 'her'. He was especially angry as Balint wrote about some of Beba's most intimate feelings.

Henry was very independent minded, and he and Beba strongly believed in the therapeutic effect of an injection of Synacthen for a variety of medical conditions. Synacthen is adrenocorticotrophic hormone. Its effect is to increase steroid blood levels produced by the adrenal glands.

I was very reluctant to administer this as I could find no evidence about its use. They were using it for backache, migraines, and all sorts of other conditions. I had one patient who had severe psoriasis who pleaded with me to give him a Synacthen injection as it worked a year previously. I

---

[17]   Michael Balint. 1957. *The Doctor, His Patient and the Illness*. Churchill Livingstone.

gave him one injection and his psoriasis completely cleared and his skin remained in a good condition for the next six months. Synacthen is now used for such conditions as rheumatoid arthritis, ulcerative colitis, and infantile spasms but its effect may be short lived.

My mother retired as a GP in 1975 but had been unable to sell her house and surgery (Tieve Tara). Kath and I had been house-hunting, and we found we simply could not afford a house at London prices. One day, on impulse, we decided to approach my mother and offer to buy her house and surgery and set up a general practice there. I had decided working in Roehampton was not for me. My mother sold us the house at a generously low price, and Kath was willing to give up her really good consultancy job in London. This was a really big sacrifice for Kath for which I am eternally grateful.

CHAPTER 8

GENERAL PRACTICE IN CASTLEFORD

Castleford is situated ten miles north-east of Wakefield. The city of Wakefield is the site of both the metropolitan district council and the administrative bodies for the NHS. The Wakefield district has a population of about 350,000 and Castleford about 36,000.

Castleford was a mining town with three flourishing coal mines. All three were closed after the miners' strike in 1984/5. This partly resulted in unemployment rising to over 20 per cent.

Airedale is a suburb of Castleford and is one of the most deprived areas in the UK.

The NHS used to grade areas according to the need for GPs. Castleford was, in 1978, designated an 'open' area. That meant a doctor was allowed to set up in practice after simply submitting an application to the Family Practitioner Committee (FPC). That meant Castleford was under-doctored. After I started working there, the area became 'intermediate' so that special conditions had to be met before another GP could be taken on. The third classification was 'closed' and a very special case had to be made for taking on an extra GP. I mentioned Maureen and Paddy in Chapter 1. They were the daughters of Mrs McGrath, my parents' housekeeper. Paddy's husband, Ernest, was a builder. We had the house and surgery decorated, and Ernest undertook these alterations. We organised all this from London by telephone.

We were to start on 1 November 1978. Kath took charge of the administration and was the practice manager. The government reimbursed the practice with 70 per cent of staff salaries. However, this was not allowed for wives of GPs. She worked for a number of years without pay until the rules were changed. However, she was contributing to our income with her work. To do this and give up her London job was truly selfless.

On that day, we had a fully equipped surgery with two consulting rooms, a waiting room, and a reception room but no patients.

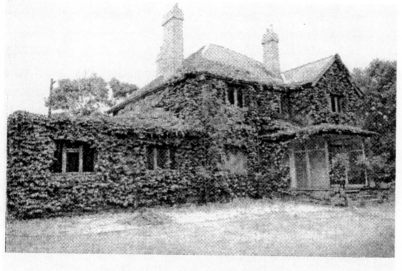

"Tieve-Tara (The House on the Hill) 1978"

Tieve Tara 1978

The surgery is the single-story extension to the private house and was approached separately by an unsurfaced rough track. The house was approached by a private drive that also served six neighbouring properties.

At that time, the NHS regulations made it very difficult for a patient to change GP. Every person in the UK had a medical card on which there is registered the name of their GP. A lot of patients lost these cards. Indeed, I was one of those. If they could find their medical card, it had to be taken to their existing GP to get a signature to give permission to change doctor. This could have been embarrassing. Then it took two weeks for the patient to become registered after handing in the medical card. However, one could be registered immediately if the address had changed. I took advice. One could register a patient immediately if he or she signed a statement to the effect that they did not wish to obtain the signature of their last GP. None of the Castleford GPs at that time were accepting patients who wanted to change doctor. I was very unpopular, of course, as the main way I could build up a practice was for patients coming from another general practice. This resulted in that practice losing income. There was no problem with patients moving into the area from another place.

At 9.25 a.m. on that 1 November, my first patient arrived. I gave him a really thorough examination (he had a cold). Of course, I wanted him to go away and spread the word as to how good we were. I had a significant number of old friends who not only joined the list but also spread the word. These included the Goodenough family, Peter and Judith Box, the Wheeldons and the Doncasters. Mrs May Wheeldon J. P. was a friend of my parents and was a great help. I mentioned Grahame Smith in Chapter 2. He was a fellow medical student and flatmate when we were at University College. He married Caroline (who was a nurse at the London Hospital) and he became a GP working in Pontefract, which is four miles from Castleford. They became two of my first patients, and on the day of their registration, Caroline announced to me that she was pregnant. She wanted a home delivery. I knew I would be a nervous wreck about that when the time came. Kath and I became patients of Grahame's practice.

I had been advised that I should approach this venture as though was setting up a new retail shop. I must have a product better than the other shops and do things differently. In 1978, there was a great reluctance for GPs to visit patients at home. I did the opposite and anyone who asked, I visited. I was not allowed by some of the other GPs to use the out-of-hours deputising service. I worked for two months without any time off whatsoever.

I was desperate to get some help especially at weekends. I advertised for weekend help in the medical journals and local newspapers. I got one early reply, which was written in pencil on a scrap of lined paper. The address was S. Royds Hospital. This was the local psychiatric hospital. The application was obviously a hoax and the applicant maintained that one asset for the job was that he had a 'weak end'. The other was that he worked in the mortuary and so knew how to talk to patients properly. The letter turned out to be from my uncle Sam, who had been a GP in Wakefield until he retired to Northern Ireland. He had *The Wakefield Express* posted to him each week. My advert was in that paper each week for about a month. The only other enquiry I had was from a married couple working in Pontefract Hospital. They helped me out at weekends despite being very busy in their posts at the local hospital in Pontefract. Drs Anne Martin and Ted McGrath are truly good people, and I am eternally grateful to them. I offered Anne a partnership but she decided to work in Hemsworth and then Pontefract. Later, for about a year, I went into an out-of-hours rota with Grahame Smith's practice. That was a very kind act of that practice. The senior partner of that practice was John Waring. One Saturday I became ill from stress, and he came to see me as my GP. He insisted on my stopping work. We could not find anyone to stand in for me so he took over himself. This was a truly altruistic act. I got back from a holiday, and there was a letter informing me that a proper out-of-hours service was starting, which was to be manned by local GPs and the three directors were Drs Graeme Slack, Phillip Earnshaw, and Martin Johnson. I could have kissed each one of them.

My pay cheque at the end of December 1978 was £2.96 less 6 per cent pension contribution. The reason for that is explained by the method GPs were paid at that time. The number of registered patients was counted on the first of each quarter, that is, January, April, July, and October. I started on 1 November. On 1 October, I was not there and had no patients on my list. The £2.96 was for taking a cervical smear and was an item of service payment. At the end of my first year, the gross income was £7,567, but after paying wages and other expenses, the practice made a loss of £3,048. Fortunately, Kath and I owned a flat in Devon, which we sold. This enabled us to have a decent lifestyle. However, it was vital that the practice became viable in the second year or we would have to leave.

General practices directly employed staff such as the practice manager, receptionists, and a practice nurse. Seventy per cent of the salary of directly employed staff was reimbursed to the practice. There was also attached staff employed by the health authority, local hospital, or other bodies. These included the health visitors and midwife.

In 1979, Kath left the practice to first set up her own catering business and later took on the job as manager of Nostel Priory Enterprises. Nostel Priory is our local stately home. Kath returned as practice manager in 1986.

In 1979, we employed Joyce Hunt as a secretary/receptionist and Anne Long as a receptionist. Joyce was an excellent shorthand typist who refused to use an electric typewriter. Kath provided her with her mother's manual typewriter. Joyce's husband, Ken, walked our dog for us when he was not working and when Kath and I were busy. He was a West Riding bus driver. We offered patients the service of having their repeat prescriptions prepared for collection at the local pharmacy of their choice. There were several pharmacies on the main street of Castleford town, two miles from Tieve Tara. Ken delivered the prescriptions for us from his bus first thing each morning. Just before Joyce retired, she was inputting summaries of patient records on to a sophisticated computer system.

Anne had a chronic illness and was a truly loyal receptionist. She would work at home for us when she was too ill to come to work. She died in her early thirties. It was a tragedy.

The core attached staff at that time comprised district nurses, health visitor, and midwives. The problem for the administrative bodies was how to decide how much attached staff input there should be with such a small practice. Obviously I had to share attached staff with other practices, which was fine. Larger practices had their own attached staff working solely for them. Sister Margaret Ellis was the district nurse and was particularly skilled at looking after terminally ill patients. When the practice had its first pregnant woman I was allocated a senior midwife, Sister Joyce Pearson. We held an antenatal clinic once a fortnight. Occasionally the patient did not turn up so we had a good old gossip. I was indeed a nervous wreck when the time came for my friend Caroline to deliver Amy. I went into the maternity department at Pontefract Hospital to check the equipment and made sure I had all the necessary drugs. One morning just before I was about to start my surgery, I had a phone call from Sister Pearson that Caroline had had a normal delivery and all was well. What a relief!

The practice was provided with a full-time health visitor at a very early stage. Sue Smith had great expertise with non-accidental injury of babies (child abuse), and we discovered that the practice had attracted a very high number of cases and potential cases. Single-handed practice is lonely for the GP, and I was under a lot of stress. Kath was my main soulmate and comforter. Sue was a very significant medical soulmate and she became my patient and our friend to this day. She later obtained a Ph.D. and runs her own successful business.

The practice patients were certainly deprived and more deprived than the patients of neighbouring practices. This was because they received more time from me when the practice was very small. At that time, a practice in a deprived area received the same funding as one in a more affluent area. Over the years, I got to know colleagues working in the more affluent areas and could compare notes. Ackworth near Pontefract was one of these contrasting practices. We had often had to write more than one letter to a woman inviting her to come in for a smear. Ackworth had to turn down requests from women asking for their smears early.

In the early 1980s, we employed a second receptionist, Andrea Woodward. In 2012, she is still working in the new medical centre, and she has been there the longest of any of the directly employed staff.

As the number of patients built up, I found the workload increasingly stressful and my mother came out of retirement to help me. She became an equity partner. There was a clause in her last partnership agreement with Dr Suniel Minocha that after retirement she was not allowed to work within a five-mile radius of Tieve Tara Surgery. This was a standard clause in all GP partnership agreements at that time. There was much debate as to whether this would stand up in law. One evening I was in our kitchen and the doorbell rang. It was a man from a solicitor's office who served an injunction on the practice requiring me to close it forthwith. I informed the FPC first thing the next morning. The FPC made arrangements with Dr Minocha and another neighbouring practice to look after the patients until I reopened. I put a notice on the surgery door to inform the patients. The reason for the injunction was my mother breaking the clause in her partnership agreement mentioned above. There was a court case and my mother was not allowed to work for me. She had to pay a fine, legal costs, and Dr Minocha's expenses (which included the cost of a cup of tea). He was in partnership with his wife, Devica Minocha. I have had a warm professional relationship with her throughout that time and to the present day. Suniel Minocha died at the age of 76 in 2004.

Holidays are a problem and an expense for a single-handed GP. A locum has to be employed. One locum we had was a trainee GP from Cheltenham. My mother, who was not allowed to practise at Tieve Tara Surgery, supervised him. That certainly would not be allowed at this time. Some of the locums we used were terrible, and we received lots of complaints from the patients. Even when you were abroad on holiday, you were responsible for the actions of a locum. This changed later such that a locum was responsible for his or her own actions. Other locums were excellent. John Papworth-Smith was one such. I employed him as an assistant/locum to both work with me and be a locum for a holiday. He did things over and above what was expected of him. I suffered from recurrent perianal abscesses. I had one particularly bad one and was unable to sit down without excruciating pain. Shortly before a surgery, he incised the abscess to drain the pus. He did this on my couch in our lounge. I was then able to do the surgery. On another occasion, my mother became ill and required a hospital admission.

John drove her to the hospital, and I did the surgery. I offered him a partnership but he decided to continue as a GP for the University of Leeds. No one seemed to want to work with me!

Since my experience of teaching undergraduates and of some postgraduate education in Cheltenham, I decided to approach Leeds Medical School to see whether I could be involved with the teaching of medical students. John Lee came for a couple of weeks and was a breath of fresh air. In 1983, I advertised for a partner and, in contrast to the advert for weekend help, received about ninety applications. We had applied for permission to extend the surgery and that was an attraction. I was also planning to become a trainer of GPs. I interviewed about five doctors and one of them was Dr John Lee. In the end, I offered him the job for two reasons. The first was that he was the only one who knew how difficult the area was. The second was because he was so nice to our dog. I was also impressed that he was the only applicant who had private medical insurance. The reason he gave for that was he wanted to take as little time off work as possible. I had to take a huge drop in salary to take on a partner but it was worth it. There was an out-of-hours service, and I could have every other night off duty during the week. John joined us in 1984.

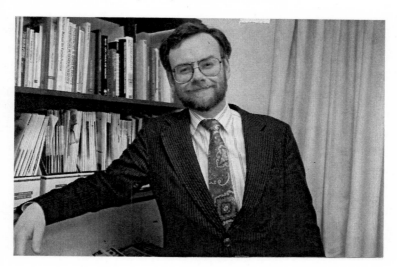

John Lee.

I was determined to be a trainer of prospective GPs. I thought that there would be a rule introduced that all trainers should have passed the examination of MRCGP (Member the Royal College of General Practitioners). I had failed this on my first attempt while I was in Cheltenham. I argued with an examiner in the oral exam. That was not a wise thing to do, but to this day I believe he was definitely wrong. After I was settled in Yorkshire, I decided I would keep taking the examination until I passed it. It actually did me a favour as I had to get up to date, which was difficult as a single-handed GP. I sat the examination in 1984. There was a multiple choice paper. I hated multiple choice questions. I think I analysed the choices too deeply. I very much doubted I had passed.

The written parts were taken in Leeds and the viva in London. Again I rebelled, but this time in the written section. How stupid can one be? One part of the examination asked for notes to be written. I was an essay man. I wrote essays. One of the essays I wrote was on the Black Report. This was published in 1980 and was about health and social deprivation. The only thing I knew about it was from a ten-minute item on the BBC's *Newsnight* programme. You can see from the writing in this chapter that I can be somewhat verbose. I wrote at length on the Black Report. I thought I had definitely failed. The viva went well this time.

The results were sent by post but published a day earlier on a viewdata system called Prestel. I knew that a travel agent in Castleford used Prestel, so I persuaded them to look up the examination results. All those who passed were listed alphabetically. The travel agent started at the letter A, and there was a very slow scroll down the alphabet. Eventually my name appeared and I was ecstatic. I remained composed until I was outside in the street and then I punched the air and shouted out loud.

I describe the process of becoming a trainer and my experiences in postgraduate general practice education in the next chapter.

A trainee is supposed to be supernumerary, but he or she is definitely an extra pair of hands after learning the ropes. They shared the visits and could be on call with one of us supervising. I used to wind John Lee up about the trainees. For example, when Andrew Sykes was about to start as a trainee, I told John about Andrew's degree in genetics. John was anxious we would get a trainee who knew more than he or I. This did not bother me.

There was money available for us to extend the surgery building into some of our garden. This turned out to be a really good investment for Kath and me. Kath and I sold part of the garden to me and John Lee for the same amount we had paid my mother for the five-bedroom house and surgery. Our private house had therefore cost us nothing. The extension allowed each partner to have a consulting room, and there was also one for the trainee and practice manager. There was a small common room, which contained the library of books and journals required of a training practice.

The patient numbers slowly but surely increased as did our income. Eventually, wives of GPs were allowed to be paid and have the 70 per cent reimbursement like anyone else. Kath, John, and I held partners' meetings in the kitchen of our house, and we usually started with a gin and tonic. This felt very civilised. GPs are generally self-employed businessmen, and Kath was in effect a managing director. The meetings had an agenda, and minutes were taken.

Our second trainee, Anne Godridge, enjoyed working with us so much that when she had completed her GP training she approached us to see whether we could possibly take her on as a partner. This was a bit of a shock as we had not grown enough for a full third partner. It would involve John and I taking a significant drop in salary. However, we worked something out, and Anne started part-time. It was a great decision. I had heard from Jean Wharton, a consultant physician at Pontefract, that Anne had the best bedside manner of any doctor she had come across. I knew that from being her trainer. I also knew she had a great sense of humour. Anne, John, Kath, and I made a great team, and the practice went from strength to strength.

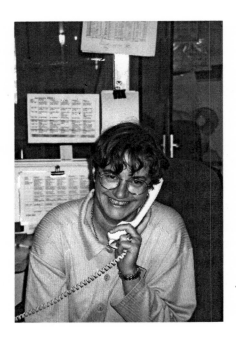

Anne Godridge.

We soon became cramped for space, and the surgery was once more enlarged. The financial situation regarding surgery buildings was complex. A loan was taken out from a body called the General Practice Finance Corporation (GPFC). There was then a calculation based partly on what rent one could realise if the premises were let on a commercial basis. The government paid us a 'cost rent'. This money generally covered repayments to the GPFC. The loan included costs such as architects' and solicitors' fees. There were strict NHS rules as to the area of waiting, consulting, and other rooms. If one did not stick to the rules, one might not be entitled to the full cost rent. Rates were reimbursed by the government. If in the fullness of time, the loan was paid off, then this would be a very favourable investment. One could sell one's share of the building to an incoming replacement partner on retirement. There were lots of expenses of the practice, and these were allowed against tax. For example, electricity, the telephone, repairs, the cleaner, and a percentage of our cars were all legitimate expenses. We had to buy in dressings and drugs for emergency use as well as stationery. All of this came out of the gross earnings of the partners.

What was the nature of our work and the workload? Visit requests could be very heavy. We experimented with one partner undertaking the visits starting at 9 a.m. and not doing a morning surgery. This was inefficient and probably encouraged visit requests. We sometimes did twenty visits in the first half of the morning. We abandoned this experiment and many years later introduced nurse triage. This meant that any visit requests and some other problems were put through on the phone to an experienced practice nurse such as Melanie Hanney or Christine Hunter. We were one of the first practices to do this, and our work was presented to other GPs working in our area at a large education meeting. It was also presented at a national conference and published. An appointment system was introduced when John Lee became a partner. One of the requirements of a training practice was to have ten-minute appointments, which was pretty civilised. Before that, we ran open surgeries. With open surgeries, the numbers attending were unpredictable and could be many. On the other hand, appointment surgeries were always booked up, and we experimented over the years with all sorts of different systems. We did see extra patients and slotted others in between appointments. The system was properly sorted out only in the early 2000s by a new partner, Dr Sarah Baker. We worked really hard one week so that every appointment the following week was free. Some were bookable in advance and others on the day. From that day on, there were no extras to be seen at the end of a surgery.

In Airedale, there was high unemployment and high rates of long—and short-term sickness requiring certification by the GP. Many families had unhealthy diets, and there was a very significant abuse of alcohol and drugs. There were higher-than-average cases of angina, heart attacks, and chronic bronchitis. There was a high prevalence of psychiatric illness. Many patients reading this will not recognise themselves in the list of medical problems just mentioned. The majority of the patients were hard working, looking after their health, and coming to us early with any worrying symptoms. As in nearly all general practices, a significant number of patients simply did not attend the precious appointments. This could amount to three hours of lost surgery time each week.

There is not the scope in this book to describe all the medical conditions I encountered, but I will make some observations about the coal miners and their families. Before I started in Airedale, my mother had jokingly told me that all I needed to know about was athlete's foot and chest diseases. This was because coal miners commonly suffered from a fungal infection of their feet transmitted from workmates in the shower rooms at the pit. There was lots of smoking, as well as pneumoconiosis from the dust in the mines. As I mentioned in Chapter 1, Fryston Village is within walking distance of our house and the surgery. Fryston Colliery was the main feature of Fryston Village. In the early 1980s, it employed about 1,500 men. The adjacent Fryston Village had houses mainly occupied by miners but not exclusively. I got to know a lot of the miners and their families there very well. They were tough and could be described as salt of the earth. (Jack Hulme, photographer, lived there and has captured Fryston life in one of his books.[18] He is reported as having taken 10,000 photographs of Fryston. He used to come up to our house and take photographs at my birthday parties when I was a child. (He was our photographer at the opening of the first extension to the surgery). The Fryston Hotel was a large pub just outside Fryston at the bottom of the private drive to our house. Serious beer drinking went on there by the miners and their partners. Our neighbour, Martin Raftery was a retired miner from Fryston, and he organised a gang of us from the surgery to go down Fryston Colliery. It was seven miles to the place where coal was cut (the coalface), and we travelled part of the way on a coal belt and the rest on a small railway. It was very hot, and when I emerged I was incredibly thirsty, the dirtiest I had ever been, and with backache from bending so much. I could empathise with the miners who were unable to work for periods of time because of what might be perceived as minor illnesses. I could also understand why they quenched their thirst after work in the Fryston Hotel.

---

18   World Famous Round here: The photographs of Jack Hulme. Jack Hulme, Richard van Riel, Olive Fowler, Harry Maltkin. Yorkshire Art Circus in Association with Wakefield Metropolitan District Council. 1990.

I gave out medical certificates of unfitness to work to miners very easily. There were injuries down the pit and one of my coal miner patients was killed. I had another couple of families who had lost the father of the household in fatal pit accidents. There were many cases of chronic bronchitis and emphysema (destroyed areas of the lung from infection and the pressure of coughing). Coal miners' pneumoconiosis is caused by long-term exposure of the lungs to coal dust. Both the latter and progressive emphysema lead to breathlessness, which can be very distressing and life threatening. Pontefract General Infirmary had an excellent chest unit headed by consultant chest physician Michael Peake. As I describe in Chapter 9, I worked closely with Mick Peake on education matters. He and our MP, Sir Geoffrey Lofthouse, now Lord Lofthouse (who was himself a coal miner in his youth), fought for years to get emphysema in coal miners recognised as an industrial disease and attract compensation. They eventually succeeded. Pneumoconiosis already was such an industrial disease. The level of compensation awarded after death was determined by a post-mortem to which the miner had committed himself in writing. Sometimes the family did not know about this, and this did not help when dealing with the bereaved.

The miners' strike of 1984/5 created some specific medical problems. There were more children to see in the surgery because the fathers panicked somewhat and would not let the mothers leave things for a while to see whether there was an improvement with time. Lots of miners came to us with symptoms of depression and other conditions, and we gave out lots of sickness certificates. This helped with their finances. I had one miner who had lost weight because he could not chew properly because of a terrible toothache. He could not afford to go to a dentist. Families became very close, and there was a fantastic supporting spirit in Airedale. The local shopkeepers helped out as best as they could. There is no through road in Fryston, and a picket line was set up at the entrance to the village to prevent any miner going to work. They had a hut and a brazier to keep them warm through the cold winter's nights. Ian MacGregor was the head of the National Coal Board at the time, and the picket hut had very rude words about him and the prime minister, Margaret Thatcher.

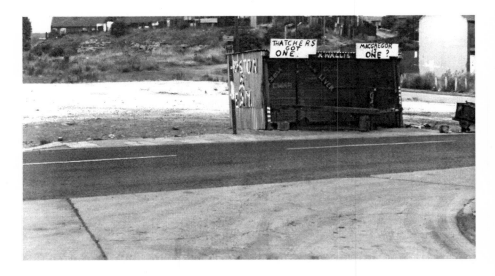

Picket hut.

John Lee and I had to drive through the picket line to get to home visits. I always stopped and asked, 'Can I go and get some coal out of that pit?' I was always told, 'Of course, help yourself'. I took a bottle of whisky down to them one evening. Towards the end of the strike, the picket line was manned by men from another area. We were awakened one night by the noise of a violent clash between these men and the police. Apparently, this noise was louder than anything that had occurred in the Second World War. The latter part of the 1980s and first half of the 1990s were grim in Castleford with closure of all the Castleford coal mines and high unemployment. There was also a lack of jobs generally in the UK.

Heroin addiction became a major problem in Airedale. Anne, John, and I started to manage these patients in the surgery. Very few practices in the district were willing to undertake this work in the 1980s. Over the years, Anne became trained up for this special work and started working in a dedicated clinic run by Turning Point. (Turning Point was founded in 1964 in London as an alcohol project. It developed into a large social care organisation dealing with drug abusers among other things). At one time we were looking after about sixty addicts and their families. New cases joined our list when it got around that we were helping. Prescriptions for the replacement therapy, methadone, had to be written by hand in a specific way on a special blue prescription sheet. This took up significant time. The practice was not paid extra for this work. The behaviour of some of these patients was sometimes bad. Sitting on the floor in the corridor and sleeping in the waiting room was common. I made the mistake of leaving one such patient in my consulting room while I went to reception to get something. On my return, I noticed a large bulge under his pullover. I stared at it and he burst into tears producing our video camera he was intending to steel. He genuinely apologised to me and asked me to forgive him. I said I would do nothing about this and continued with the consultation. In 1996, John Lee resigned and took up jobs in dermatology and genito-urinary medicine. He was sorely missed. He was replaced by Mohan Bazaz, who eventually pointed out to us the disruptive influence of our drug abusers. Some of them were very demanding on the receptionists and doctors. We decided that their management should be taken over by the Turning Point clinics. We would continue to issue prescriptions for them. We had to be very tough with those who wanted their prescriptions early. The whole family was usually affected, and there were significant associated mental health problems. In those years our house was broken into on two occasions while we were in bed. Valuable antiques were left but such things as a video player or camera were stolen. These were sold and the money used to feed their drug habit for a day or two. It is a dreadful feeling to have one's home violated in such a way.

This experience hardened my belief in maintenance therapy with methadone. Maintenance therapy is sticking to roughly the same dose of methadone each day and not attempting a withdrawal. We worked with other patients who wanted to withdraw. We all knew that the maintenance approach reduced crime in the area and actually saved a lot of money in police time.

In 1999, because of Anne's work, the practice was awarded Beacon status by the government. We were very proud of that.

In 1991, the Conservative Government introduced GP fundholding. The scheme provided GP practices with monies from which to purchase hospital and other services such as physiotherapy. The calculation of the fund was complicated, and any moneys saved by the practice could be reinvested into equipment or the surgery building. Generally, equipment and the building were owned by the partners. A partner therefore could cash in on leaving. Alternatively, the partnership could make a profit by selling the buildings on to a private company and then paying rent. Holding back on referring patients to a hospital consultant or issuing cheaper medicines could result in great savings. In my opinion then and now, the whole think stank and was unethical. The partnership joined an anti-fundholding group of like-minded practices called 'The five towns' family doctors' forum'. We were obviously losing out financially and the last straw was when our community psychiatric nurse, Mark Barker, was moved to a neighbouring fundholding practice. He was not replaced. The members of the multifund were eventually forced by the health authority to become fundholders. Our practice was too small to go it alone with fundholding so we partnered Douglas Diggle's practice in South Elmsall (fifteen miles away). His practice was of a similar size. We had a computer dedicated to working out the fundholding situation in a corner of the surgery. Someone from the health authority came in and analysed the data relevant to the scheme. We largely ignored the fundholding scheme. Once a year, Douglas Diggle and I met Wendy Pearson, a senior manager from the health authority. She was the finance administrator of the fundholding scheme. The object of the meeting was for us to go through the fundholding finances. We had no idea what she was talking about and simply nodded at appropriate times. Eventually we were allowed to go it alone and again we largely ignored the scheme. Other practices embraced fundholding with open arms. I discovered during attendance allowance (see later) examinations that patients were not being referred to consultants by some of my GP colleagues. The chief executive of the health authority in the years before the 1997 general election was Keith Salisbury. At that time, the health authority had a significant financial deficit, and he visited each practice requesting a financial contribution from fundholding savings. I got my wallet out and offered to give him £5. He was a charming man but did not charm me. At a meeting for GPs before the 1997 election, he assured those present that fundholding was 'set in' and could not be abolished as the Labour Party were promising. The year 1997 saw Tony Blair's landslide election result and fundholding was abolished in 1998.

Our practice manager, Kath, took us through the Kings Fund Organisational Audit in 1994/5. This involved writing up policies and procedures after an initial detailed checklist had been undertaken. The checklist might, for example, reveal that we had no written procedure for dealing with repeat prescription requests or no policy for dealing with the press. We had to have a policy for dealing with riots. There were many areas of our work to be visited and the process took well over a year. We were helped by Julia Taylor, a King's Fund Audit facilitator, employed by the health authority. We had to put everything together in a manual and present this before an inspection of the practice was made. The inspection was by an external team that included a GP. The GP was from the East End of London and understood full well what it was like to work in a deprived area. We got together with other practices who were taking part in the scheme, and there was some extra funding provided. We felt very proud when we passed the inspection. It had been a great team achievement.

Kath then facilitated the team in a project that resulted in the practice obtaining the Investors in People award. The partners at the time were Anne, Mohan Bazaz, and I. At a partners' meeting to discuss Investor in People, Kath put the question to us 'Are you aware of the principles of Investors in People?' We all answered yes. She then said 'Well, what are they?' We had no idea! She then explained them to us in detail. Investors in People looks for leadership qualities, teamwork, continuing learning and training, rewarding good work, career development, involving patients, and so on. Like the King's Fund Organisational Audit, the process is completed by a visiting inspector who chooses a selection of people to interview one to one. Our inspector was Viv, who we had heard was very tough. We were all very nervous. The first person she interviewed was Madge, our cleaner. Madge was a forthright speaker who stood for no-nonsense from anyone. Madge closed the door firmly behind her and said in a loud voice, 'Right. What does tha want?' When

Viv reported back, she told us how impressed she was with Madge and her loyalty. We were very proud when we received our award.

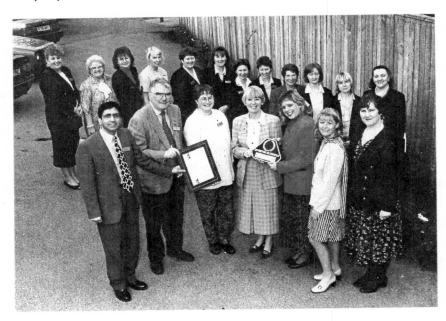

The Investors in People award. Back row: Hazel Bird, Madge Charlesworth, Lynn Armstrong, Margaret Wilks, Jean Stones, Janet Pease, Jean Howarth, Andrea Woodward, Irene Nickleson, Christine Hunter, Jackie Spencer, Kathryn Padget. Front Row: Mohan Bazaz, I, Anne Godridge, Kath, and three women from the Investor in People Organisation.

We had a great team in the surgery. Indeed we held several teambuilding events over the years at significant expense to the practice. One such event involved an overnight stay in the smart Waterton Park Hotel. Sometimes we had an outside facilitator and others we facilitated ourselves.

We had a bad experience when we were looking for a replacement partner for John Lee. Anne (alto), I (tenor), and John (bass and pianist) were all members of the Castleford Choral Society. The advert in the *British Medical Journal* read something like 'Tenor and Alto require additional singer to become a partner ...' We had one reply who applied in a similar tone. He had an ideal curriculum vitae. We interviewed him and offered him the job. We held a celebratory party for him and the whole team at our house. Just before Kath and I were to holiday in the USA, he wrote changing his mind and telling us he felt we were too familiar with the staff. We were very angry indeed. In New Orleans, I bought a voodoo doll and pins. When we got back from holiday, I put the doll and pins in reception with a note, 'Think of someone you met at a party recently and use the pins accordingly'. After I had completed my appointments, I went into the reception area and found that the majority of the pins were stuck into the groin of the doll. Hazel Bird, our senior receptionist, later remarked to me, 'And didn't you even feel the slightest twinge?'

Being a training practice brought in extra money. All the partners in the 1990s earned extra by undertaking mobility and attendance allowance examinations. One was not allowed to undertake these medicals on one's own patients. If a patient had difficulty with walking, he or she might be entitled to a mobility allowance. Some of the patients could be assessed in our surgery and others had to be assessed in their home. The attendance allowance was for patients who had to have significant help and care with their daily living. These assessments were undertaken at home. We had significant training surrounding these medicals, but I felt that the government-employed doctors biased the training towards our turning patients down for these benefits.

The assessments could take well over an hour and we did them in our spare time. It was a rare opportunity to spend significant time with a patient and explore their problems in detail. With our regular GP work, it could take several ten-minute appointments to look at anything in depth. Of course we knew that some of the applicants exaggerated their problems and others knew some of the questions that they would be asked. One had to assess the speed and distance a patient could walk for the mobility allowance. This was really difficult even if one observed the patient walking for a short distance. The disability living allowance was brought in for those under sixty-five years of age. It has a mobility and care element. (I was amused by one of my patients running up the street to me to tell me he had applied for a mobility allowance). The attendance allowance was for those over sixty-five years of age. These benefits attracted significant extra income, and the mobility allowance could be used to supply a new car every few years. At the time of writing, the attendance allowance is £73.60 a week if the patient requires care during both the day and the night. In the end, the government insisted that each year we had five days of training on these benefits. This was nearly as much training I undertook for my other work as a GP. We stopped doing these medicals mainly because of the training commitment but also because the pay was not very good.

Kath had taken us through a second extension of the surgery and she retired on New Year's Eve, 1999. The practice gave her a Labrador dog as a leaving present. She called him Ben. She had a great relationship with the staff some of whom go out for lunch together regularly at the time of writing. If it were not for Kath, a lot of people would not have had jobs at Tieve Tara.

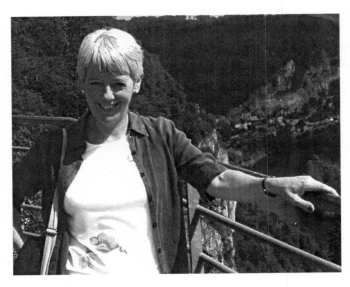

Kath.

We advertised for a practice development manager. We had a significant number of applicants and Celia Burnhope was appointed. She had considerable experience of the NHS.

The Blair government introduced primary care groups (PCGs) in 1999. Each practice had a GP member of a PCG and the area it covered was relatively small. Ours covered Castleford and Normanton. I enjoyed meeting my colleagues regularly and getting to know them better. The PCG's aim was to improve patient care. Our health visitor, Kathryn Padgett, and I co-chaired the organisational development subgroup. In 2002, PCGs were replaced by primary care trusts (PCTs). Ours was called the Eastern Wakefield PCT. It was responsible for primary care in Pontefract, Hemsworth, Featherstone, Castleford, Normanton, Ferrybridge, and other conurbations. It was responsible for commissioning hospital care as well as many other services. Many people, including me later, were employed by the PCT to improve patient care. In 2007, that PCT merged with the Western Wakefield PCT, which served Wakefield and environs. At the end of March 2013, PCTs will be abolished and replaced by clinical commissioning groups. This is a travesty.

In 1998, after fundholding was abolished, a new payment method was introduced for general practice. This was the Personal Medical Service (PMS) scheme. It was voluntary and one had to apply. It was an alternative GMS (General Medical Services) payment scheme based on the Red Book of Statement of Fees and Allowances. Most practices in our area joined the PMS scheme. Celia negotiated our PMS contract with the health authority. Because of the severe deprivation in Airedale, we obtained funding for four-and-a-half whole-time-equivalent GPs. We were three in 1998 with just over 5000 patients. There were also extra monies to pay for more practice nurses and administrators. Mohan Bazaz retired due to ill health, and we eventually had a partnership consisting of Anne, Jyoti Agawala, Sarah Baker, and I. Sarah left to become the manager of our out-of-hours service. Jyoti resigned and the partnership at the time of my retirement also included Monica Smith, Rosario Vega, and Deborah Hewitt (my last trainee). Christine Hunter had been the practice nurse for many years and was joined by Nicki Harrison. Christine successfully achieved a B.Sc. in nursing while working at our practice. This was a great achievement as she had a husband and three daughters as well as her job. Lynn Armstrong was trained up to be a health-care assistant. Jane Herbert was taken on as practice administration manager and Jean Howarth trained up from being a receptionist to become Jane's deputy.

The practice became cramped for space. We made a big decision in the absence of the practice manager. Celia was enjoying a holiday and the partners decided that she should be moved out of her office to a portacabin! Actually, the portacabin provided better conditions for her than her surgery office. We also moved the practice library to another portacabin.

The partners decided to invest in a huge extension. We formed a limited company called Motorstep Ltd. The directors and equal shareholders were Jyoti, Anne, Monica, Deborah, Celia, Christine, and I. Our spouses became shareholders later but not directors. I insisted that our practice nurse Christine should be involved because of her many years of loyal work in the practice. It seemed right only when several of the other directors had only been with us for a relatively short time. There were many meetings with architects, interviewing builders and dealing with surveyors, our solicitor, and accountant. Planning permission was granted and eventually building work started.

The building was completed in 2003 and cost about £1,800,000. It is vast. There were about twenty consulting rooms, a huge waiting room, an education suite with a room that could be used as a boardroom, a minor surgery unit, and a common room.

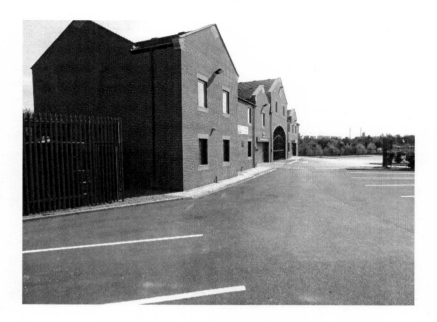

Tieve Tara medical Centre, 2003.

The day we moved in, Monica suggested we could hire out the waiting room for wedding receptions. I did not like my consulting room half as much as the one in the old building, which overlooked our private house's garden. My new room overlooked the car park, and I could never open the blind of my window. We met less often that when we used to congregate in the reception area of the old surgery. The practice received a rent from the government that just about covered the interest and capital repayments on the bank loan. Motorstep was sold to Health Investments Ltd in 2008 for over two million pounds. There was much haggling about what we were owed and one aspect of the contract had to go to arbitration, which we won. We made a reasonable profit considering the share in Motorstep Ltd cost each director £1. However, I hated the ruthlessness of big business and vowed never to get involved with anything like that again. Certainly, our solicitor, Roy Cusworth, and accountant, Nick Cudmore, earned their fees.

General practices are small businesses dealing with significant amounts of money. All practices have an accountant and a solicitor. Our accountant,

Nick Cudmore, worked for us since the start of my partnership with John Lee with whom he was a friend. Most GPs are not businessmen at heart, and Nick knew this only too well when he teased us about not understanding capital accounts after he had explained this to us annually for about twenty years. Kath set up one of the area's first Patient Participation Groups for the practice.

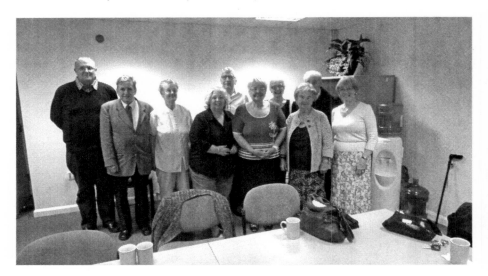

The Patient Participation Group.

The photograph is of some of the group that was still in existence at the time of my retirement. It was taken in 2011. Absent are the late Maud Raftery and also Phyllis Gaborak. It was taken in 2011. From left to right: Front—Norman Ward, Mary Bell, Margaret Baker, Jean Jordan, Pat Smith, Kath Sloan. Back: Phil Begley, Graham, Viv Williams, and Ronnie Foulkes. It was an active group that undertook surveys of patients, met regularly, and certainly had ideas to improve patient care. In 2003, the group put on a surprise party for me to celebrate my twenty-five years in the practice. What a great party we had! They published a book called *Born to Be a Doctor*, which has photos of my family and contributions from the patients who were in the group. It was a wonderful thing to do for my family.

Kath and the partners ensured that we were generous with the staff when it came to parties, particularly at Christmas. The alcohol flowed freely and we all had great fun.

A new contract for GPs was introduced in 2004, and the main feature of this was the Quality and Outcome Framework (QOF). This was a set of standards and targets for which if achieved attracted points. The maximum points that could be attained were 1,050. For each point, there was a payment to the practice of £77.50. Thus maximum points attracted a huge amount of extra income for the partnership. I felt that achieving these targets definitely improved patient care and prevented complications of illnesses. The starting point for a lot of the targets was to have a list of, for example, all diabetics, heart attack cases, patients with high blood pressure, and those with severe mental illness. Take diabetes as an example. All diabetics had to have a measure of their blood HbA1C levels. The lower this is, the better the control of their blood sugar. More points were awarded for the best controlled diabetics. There was therefore an incentive to review diabetics thoroughly and help advise them how to achieve better control, which can only be a good thing. At the review of a diabetic, one went through a checklist, which included examination of the eyes, assessment of the circulation in the feet, cholesterol level, and so on. All this information was entered into a template on the patient's computer record. There was a sophisticated software programme that analysed the results and informed how one was doing collecting QOF points. The whole practice team was involved with QOF, particularly the nurses. QOF was administered by the PCT, which was the body that administered primary care at that time. Once a year, the QOF status of the practice was inspected by a team of three. There was a PCT manager, GP assessor, and a layperson. These inspections took half a day, and I will go into more detail in Chapter 11, which describes my experience as one of the QOF medical assessors. QOF was modified and updated annually and is now administered by the National Institute for Health and Clinical Excellence (NICE).

When it came to our QOF inspection, I was so nervous that I remained in my consulting room. I made the excuse that I worked for the PCT and should not be involved.

Most practices in the 1970s kept patient information in Lloyd George envelopes. These were introduced in about 1911 by David Lloyd George when he was the minister of health. They are still in existence at the time of writing.

They were A5 in size and very untidy. In 1978, Kath and I decided to have the records kept in A4 folders. The great disadvantage of this was they took up at least twice the storage space. However, they were civilised and easy to use. Only one or two practices in the country had A4 records at the time and none in our district.

To become a training practice, the patient record had to be summarised so one could see at a glance the main and chronic problems of each patient. This was a big job, and we employed a health visitor to do some of these. John Lee and I did as many as we could.

I bought a computer for about £3,000 in 1980. Information was stored on disks. There was only the capacity for patients' names, addresses, and dates of birth recorded. This was the start of a computerised age/sex register. We never really progressed this as one day I accidentally erased half of the data that our receptionist Anne Long had painstakingly input.

In 1987, computer systems were offered to general practices at no cost. We opted to have the system manufactured by Meditel. By 1997, most general practices were computerised. This was a revolution for us as now we could print out prescriptions in our consulting rooms and also the large numbers of repeat prescriptions in a batch. There was a steep learning curve for us all. It took us a number of years to become paper light and then paperless. We employed people to input the patient records, summaries, and salient parts of hospital and other letters. Eventually correspondence received was scanned into patient records. Sophisticated search tools were introduced. Between 2000 and 2005, there were two very significant IT developments. The first was that investigation results were sent down the line to the practice. These were looked at on the screen by the GP who had ordered them and actions decided upon before the results sent to the patient record. The second development was the 'choose and book' system. This enables the GP to make an appointment with a consultant of the patient's choice at the hospital of his or her choice. This could be done during a consultation, if there was time, by a member of staff later, or by the patient from their home. The patient might choose an appointment that was earlier in a hospital at some distance compared with the local hospital. There was a practice Intranet with all the referral forms, policies, and procedures as well as leaflets that could be printed and handed to the patient. One could look for information with a patient using the Internet. One of the first times I looked something up with a patient was the skin condition scabies. This very itchy condition is caused by a small mite under the skin. A horrible picture was slowly revealed on the screen and this really upset the patient. I did not make that mistake again.

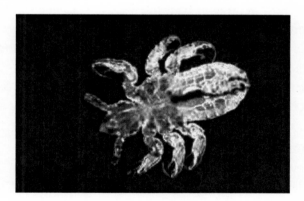

The scabies mite.

Using a computer during the consultation involved learning new skills to prevent my spending most of the consultation away from the patient and staring at a computer screen while typing.

What was it like to work in one of the most deprived areas of the United Kingdom? I mentioned earlier that we had the highest number of suspected non-accidental injury cases of any practice in the area. Case conferences took place to which the GP was invited. Very rarely did a GP attend these because they were held in surgery time. I went to as many as I could. One could really learn a huge amount about a family at one of these conferences. Invitations to the conference were sent to social workers, health visitor, the police, a solicitor, a consultant paediatrician, a consultant psychiatrist, and anyone who might be able to help make a decision about how the child and parents should be managed. Only once did I had to attend a magistrate's court about child abuse. At the end of the case, the magistrate asked the defendant mother if she had any questions. She replied, 'I would like to ask Dr Sloan what is causing this pain in my right leg'. The magistrate quickly closed the case. It was a huge responsibility to report a family with suspected child abuse, and I was lucky to have very supportive and experienced health visitors over the years, namely Susan Smith, Marjorie Robinson, Julie Barron, and Kathryn Padgett. They dealt with the children. Madeleine Davey dealt with adults. Marjorie Robinson was very experienced having been the matron of a maternity home. She was also very wise. She told me that it was her opinion that one should judge the success or otherwise of a medical activity every seven years. She died in her prime from the effects of breast cancer.

When the practice had been established and had a significant obstetric practice, Sister Pearson continued her work in Pontefract, and we were allocated Sister Mary Thornton. Mary worked with us for several years until her well-deserved retirement. She was replaced by Christine Rotherforth who was helped by Margaret Helliwell. At the time of writing, Christine had been working at Tieve Tara for twenty-five years. She is now looking after the daughters of mothers she looked after when she started. We were lucky to work with her. For a number of years, the antenatal clinics were run jointly between the midwife and the GP, the midwife seeing the mother first and then followed by an examination by the GP. I felt that all my training in obstetrics had been worthwhile. With time, maternity work was increasingly taken over by the midwives, and I felt we GPs became deskilled. I felt my role was simply to prescribe indigestion medicine when requested by the midwife. My last comment is, of course, somewhat simplistic.

John Lee and I had the largest paediatric practice in the area. We were proud of that considering neither of us had had children. Some GPs judge the development of their young patients by comparing with their own children, which is not at all good thing when working with families living in a low socio-economic environment.

There were significant behaviour problems with some of the children. One of the consultant paediatricians held her behaviour clinic on a Saturday morning and expected the GP to come along with the parents and their perceived problem child. This certainly made me focus on the most difficult problems. I attended when I was off duty often giving the family a lift in my car. From about 1990, the condition of attention deficit hyperactivity disorder was increasingly diagnosed in children older than about three. Some clinicians thought these children were simply naughty and needed discipline. The diagnosis had to be confirmed by a consultant paediatrician and part of the treatment was the prescribing of Ritalin (methylphenidate). Ritalin is a psycho-stimulant related to amphetamine. It seemed to work.

I have described how we looked after drug abusers earlier. Just before I retired, the practice started dealing with these patients in-house again. They had to be compliant and were seen by a dedicated health-care worker expert in this field. After my wife and I gave up smoking, I went to our local chemist to buy some Nicorette chewing gum. One of our heroin addicts was waiting for his methadone. He shouted across the pharmacy to me, 'Are you trying to give it up, Doc?'

Compared with some other GPs, I was very soft on the issuing of certificates for unfitness to work ('notes', called 'Lines' in Scotland). I have already mentioned this when writing about the miner's strike. One GP colleague in another part of the district was quite the opposite and told me he did not mind if a patient he had denied a certificate left his practice. Of course these patients would join a neighbouring practice where they could obtain a certificate readily. I strongly believe that a patient who is determined to get such a certificate will always succeed in the end. The Department of Health and Social Security has, for many years, employed doctors to assess those who had long-term illnesses and were certified unfit for work. Even when these doctors judged the patient to be fit for work, the patient could use the rules to obtain another certificate. A back pain case suddenly became depression. Depression became hip pain. No government will ever sort this out. I always trusted my patients and dealt with them appropriately. Doctors who persistently suspect what their patients tell them can become very bitter and cynical. However, I was most upset when one night we used a taxi and the driver was a man I had thought was totally unfit for work. I had been issuing him certificates for months. My father gave a man a certificate that stated he was fit for work. That patient then collapsed and died in my father's consulting room clutching the certificate. The certificate was quietly removed by my father who put it in his pocket.

In the 1980s and 1990s, there was significant unemployment. Some of the patients were unemployable because of lack of training and education. There is still a literacy problem to this day. Families had generations of unemployment. The unemployment situation led to depression and anxiety, which was major part of our work. We were helped by in-house community psychiatric nurses and counsellors. There was a high level of physical and verbal abuse of women. The severe and enduring mental illness cases such as bipolar disease and schizophrenia took a lot of time when there was an exacerbation. The mental health act enabled GPs to section a mental health patient (legally forcing a patient to be admitted to hospital) if a social worker and psychiatrist agreed. There were several elements of the act that enabled a section (or certification) to be for either a short or a longer time. The time could be prolonged by issuing a further certificate. The social worker was the patient advocate and on occasions disagreed with the two doctors. The patient then remained in the community. On a couple of occasions, I disagreed with the psychiatrist. A youth who had threatened a social worker with a knife and set a house on fire was in the police cells at Pontefract magistrate's court. I and the youth's solicitor as well as a senior very experienced social worker felt he should be sectioned. The psychiatrist disagreed. The psychiatrist concluded that this was a social problem. I put in a formal complaint about that consultant. Of course, nothing happened apart from the consultant ignoring me for the rest of my GP career.

My experiences with medical, surgical, paediatric, gynaecological, paediatric, dermatological, and other patients would take up too much space in a book of this nature. This chapter has been necessarily long because it covers the major part of my medical journey. That journey was peppered in the latter years by patient complaints some of which were most serious and stressful to me and my colleagues.

The majority of the complaints were dealt with according to an in-house procedure. This was written by Kath and was of such high quality that the health authority and PCT used it as a model. I had a tendency to lose my temper and say things I should not to patients. I mostly felt genuinely sorry and regretted what I had done. I often delivered the letters of apology myself and all of these patients accepted my apology and did not leave our practice. There was the case where my writing was poor on a prescription for a newborn baby. I had prescribed antibiotic eye drops, but the pharmacist had read this as ear drops which he issued to the mother. The ear drops were ten times the strength of those for the eye. I was off duty one afternoon when the surgery phoned me and told me of my mistake. I panicked and phoned Mr Prasher, a consultant ophthalmic surgeon. He heavily reassured me that there was no harm. I drove to the house and, on entering the street, saw that there was an ambulance outside the house. I panicked again. However, when I got to the house, it was a second-hand ambulance someone had bought and was using as mobile shop selling bread. What a relief! I explained things to the mother who appeared happy and gave me the registration card so her baby could be a patient of ours. However, she later went to a solicitor to pursue a complaint. My writing was indeed poor and I admitted that. She was awarded about £200. Only then did she join another practice.

There were two significant complaints in the last ten years of my GP career each involving John Lee, Anne Godridge, and me. Each of these cases took several years to come to a head. They involved our writing scores of reports and comments. The first case was heard in the Crown Court in Leeds. I had seen our Medical Defence Union (MDU) Solicitor in Manchester. He knew more medical jargon than me. I felt very confident in his opinion. The case went to the Crown Court in Leeds. The evidence was presented in a folder containing about 400 pages and called 'the bundle'. On the first day, the judge (Mrs Justice Taylor) did not speak until the late afternoon. She stopped the proceedings and said something like: 'If you turn to page 343 the word "not" should be inserted before xxxxx in line 12'. The next day she issued her verdict in legal jargon that had to be translated by our solicitor. We had won and the MDU was awarded costs. This was a civil case where the patient obtained legal aid and was seeking compensation.

The second case was again seeking compensation. It involved not only the three of us but also the Leeds and Pontefract General Infirmaries. Consideration of the evidence continued well after I had retired as a GP. A month for a court case was decided. I returned from a holiday to find a fat envelope from the MDU solicitor in Leeds. My heart sank. However, he was informing me that the case had been settled out of court. I bought a very expensive bottle of brandy and took and gave it to the solicitor to thank him. I was so relieved and could then properly enjoy my retirement.

The last patient who consulted me before I retired was my friend and colleague, Dr Grahame Smith. He was one of the very first patients who registered in 1978. In the first year as a GP in Airedale, I made an income loss of just over £3,000. In my last year as a GP, my income was just over £100,000.

The practice put on a great leaving party for me, and I was honoured that it had decided to call the learning and boardroom area of the medical centre 'The Sloan Education Suite'. I left on a high and felt very proud to have been part of Tieve Tara Medical Centre.

CHAPTER 9

GP EDUCATION AND TRAINING

An excellent history of GP training has been written by Prof. Steve Field in a chapter in a book published in 2003 by the Royal College of General Practitioners.[19] I have used his chapter to be precise about dates and an to outline the changes in the training system throughout my working life.

In 1978, the Todd Commission recommended a period of specialist training after the preclinical, clinical, and house officer training. General practice was included in this. Parliament passed an act in 1976, which made three years of vocational training mandatory in order to become a principal in general practice. This was implemented in 1982. Before that, vocational training for general practice was voluntary. I mentioned in Chapter 7 that I did not undertake any of that training but was part of the 'gold rush'.

Vocational training schemes slowly developed from the 1960s. In 1982, there were vocational training schemes in most districts of the United Kingdom. These were generally administered by staff based at a hospital's postgraduate centre. A GP (usually a trainer) worked

---

[19] Steve Field. 2003. *A Celebration of General Practice. The Story of General Practice Postgraduate Education and Training*. Chapter 10. Royal College of General Practitioners.

part-time with an administrative team. That GP post was known as the course organiser. In Yorkshire, the vocational training schemes were overseen by the deanery. The Yorkshire Deanery had various locations but eventually had a permanent base in Leeds University. In the early 1980s, the director was Dr John Sinson and his deputy Dr Jamie Bahrami.

I have already written how our practice prepared to be approved as a training practice. I had also to be approved as a trainer.

The course organiser at that time was Jeffery Ellis, a GP from Normanton. He came to my house and spent an afternoon with me in our kitchen. He explained what was required of me and smoked most of a packet of my cigarettes. He was also assessing me. He was most helpful.

There was an informal practice inspection by Dr Bahrami. This was very useful as I was not quite up to scratch. We had to buy a lot of textbooks to put in the new practice library alongside the medical books we brought from home. At that time, only training practices had libraries.

Part of the assessment involved attending a residential course. This was known as the 'O' course. I have never found out what the 'O' stood for. It was held in the College of Ripon and York St John in the city of Ripon. This was a teacher training college situated in vast grounds. The course was three days residential and run by the deanery. I was allocated a bedroom in a nearby house lived in by one of the training college teachers and his family. The course took place in a large detached Victorian building called the Short Course Centre. We ate in the college's main dining room. The food was excellent and the college had a really good wine cellar from which fine wines were served at dinner. The main facilitator of the course was Martin Rogers. It took me two days to realise he was not a doctor. He was an educationalist and we were all rather frightened of him. He was helped by a couple of course organisers. Not only were we being taught the rudiments of teaching but also we were being assessed. One had to possess appropriate knowledge, attitude, and skills to become a trainer, and at that point we were not sure what these were. It was a stressful course and there were about twenty of us from all over Yorkshire. The course started by each of us announcing our names to the group. Then the nightmare began for me. Martin Rogers insisted that each person had to remember all the others' names without writing anything down. He asked each of us to name each of the rest of the group, and when it came to me I was hopeless. That was partly because I was so anxious. After a day, one of my colleagues, Douglas Diggle, found the whole thing too much. I went for a walk with him after lunch when he told me that he was going home. He did not like the system at all and advised me to go for it and try to improve things from the inside. He did indeed leave and never became a trainer. Another colleague from Wakefield, Geoff Slater, and I decided to escape the continuous assessment of us by the course organiser tutors. We went to the other end of the complex to the students' bar and had a couple of pints of beer. After a while we half decided that the barman was a course organiser and was assessing us. Paranoia had really set in.

Martin Rogers was high powered and educational theory was a new language to us. He often split us into small groups and sent each group off to a small room to discuss something and report back to the whole group after a while. On a couple of occasions when we got to our smaller room, we had no idea what he wanted from us. Not only were taught how to teach and assess a GP trainee but also how to introduce them to working in a general practice and the record of their competence we should be making. It was a big responsibility being part of the process that eventually allows a doctor to practise independently as a GP. At the end of that course, I had no Idea how my assessment had gone but I really wanted to be a trainer.

During the previous year, I had been attending trainers' workshops that were held monthly for the trainers from the east of the Wakefield

District. I had also attended a couple of the weekly half-day teaching afternoons for the trainees. The practice passed the formal assessment by Jamie Bahrami, and the last stage of the approval process was my assessment by interview. Readers will have realised by now that I am somewhat prone to anxiety. There were about 12 interviewers, which was daunting. There was the director, deputy director, course organisers, GP tutors, and trainers. There may have been someone from the university. One prospective trainer came out after his interview and said, 'My God. They are not only asking what books you have in the practice library, they are asking what is in them!' The only thing I can remember about that interview was Dr Lutfe Kamal, a colleague from Hemsworth, greeting me at the door and leading me to my seat.

I was very pleased to get the letter informing me I had been approved as a trainer. That was in 1988. The maximum length of time for approval was three years. Just before that time expired, there was a re-inspection and reassessment of one's teaching record and skills. Attendance was expected at regular residential education courses for trainers in Ripon. Trainers were paid about £6,000 a year for their work. This I put into the practice account to contribute to the income of all the partners who had to cover for me when I was teaching.

There were about six months after the job offer when I would be allocated my first trainee. However, after about three months, I received a phone call that a trainer in another part of our area had had to stop working because of ill health. I was asked whether I could take on his trainee in three days' time. I entered a state of shock and panic.

My very first trainee was Isabel McCormick and one of the very first things she said to me was 'I don't think I want to become a GP.' The 'O' course never prepared me for that. All turned out well, and she went into general practice as her career. Indeed she came back long after she had completed her training to do a locum for Anne Godridge's maternity leave. It was a pleasure to work with her, and, like most of my trainees, we keep in touch at Christmas time. My partner, John Lee, talked in a whisper to me about anything financial because at that time Isabel's husband worked for the Inland Revenue.

Isabel was with us as a trainee for only three months. Trainees were generally attached to a general practice for six-month periods. The first trainee who was with me for the full six months was Anne Godridge. She was great fun, and when we had got to know one another, we had lots of laughs. She was born in Castleford.

At first, the trainer had to accompany the trainee to visits both in the daytime and out of hours. One of the first visits Anne and I made together was to a man with chest pain. It did not sound like a heart attack to me but Anne decided he should be admitted. He took a lot of persuading. When admitting, the GP should write an explanatory letter that is taken by the patient to the hospital. Anne did not have any writing paper and envelopes in her bag. That was a learning point. Anne also did not think the patient had had a heart attack but wanted to be sure. She was careful and was right to admit. I would not have admitted that patient. He turned out not have had a heart attack. This patient provides several teaching and discussion points and that is why I have given the case some detail here. During a later tutorial, one could explore the ethics of admitting a patient who was reluctant to go into hospital, discuss the paternalistic approach to consultations, spend time discussing what a GP should have in the emergency bag, look at what makes a high-quality letter for an admission, or compare my less careful approach and her possible defensive practice. Trainers learn a great deal from being involved in the education of trainees and students.

After I had been a trainer for ten years, the practice asked some of the trainees to make a surprise appearance at a party we were holding.

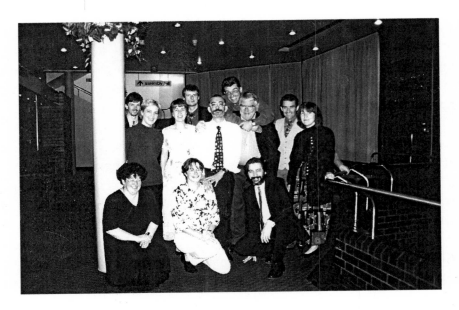

From left to right, front: Collette Coleman, Anne Godridge, Andrew Sykes. Middle: Christine Dumitrescu, Isabel McCormick, Paco Fernandez, I, Carolyn Hall. Back: Alan Kerry, Simon Acey, Norman Dawes, Simon Anderson.

I want to look at the elements of GP training at this stage rather than the personalities.

Communication and consultation skills were a vital part of the training, and it was hoped that trainees would develop a lifelong approach to improving these skills. With the written permission of patients, videos were made of consultations. These were discussed and analysed in tutorials. It was good practice for the trainer to video his or her consultations and look at them with the trainee. It was a little stressful at first having a camera in the consulting room but one soon forgot about it. I had one woman who told me on camera that the consultation she had just experienced with me was the best of her life. I think she enjoyed being filmed! We had two tutorials each week. One was based around a topic that could be a medical condition such as asthma, blood pressure, raised cholesterol, and so on. Other topics could be non-clinical such as the role of the practice manager, general practice finances, relationship with consultants, and so on. The other type of tutorial was around consultation skills. We did joint surgeries taking it in turns to observe one another's consultations. Always the experimenter, I once videoed a consultation and then videoed me and the patient watching it. The patient's comments were what I wanted to capture.

Once a month the trainers associated with Pontefract Postgraduate Centre met for an evening trainers' workshop. We discussed any problems we had with our trainees. We also looked at ways of improving our teaching skills. Jeffrey Ellis was our long-standing course organiser. He would ask one of his trainers to lead on a topic in the trainees' half-day release afternoon. Each week a whole afternoon was devoted to the trainees attending an education session in Pontefract Hospital's Postgraduate Centre.

Most large hospitals had a postgraduate centre. Pontefract's had a lecture room, a smaller teaching room, as well as some offices. There was also a comprehensive library with a librarian (Jane Smethurst). The library was for use by both the hospital doctors and those working in general practice. Jane was a fantastic help obtaining papers if one was looking into anything in depth. There were no charges for photocopying. Elsie Green was the postgraduate centre administrator. At first she had no other help. She was later joined by Pamela Wood.

I have described the process of becoming approved as a trainer. How did one become a trainee?

The training to become a GP was generally three years. A doctor who had just completed the pre-registration house officer year and was registered had two roads that could end in completion of the required training. The first was to self-construct the three years with two years of approved hospital jobs and two six-month attachments in a GP training practice. These posts could be anywhere in the UK. The second road was to apply to be accepted to work for three years in the same vocational training scheme administered by postgraduate centre people. Like the self-constructed programme, there were the same periods of hospital and GP attachments. Pontefract had such a scheme as did the postgraduate centre at Pinderfields Hospital, Wakefield. The scheme was run by the course organiser and the postgraduate centre administrative staff. Vacancies were advertised in appropriate journals and then interviews took place. At Pontefract, the interviewers consisted of the course organiser, trainers, and hospital consultants. The interviewers split into two. Applicants were therefore interviewed twice with standard questions. We were looking at attitudes as well as knowledge. There was a marking sheet that Jeffrey Ellis had designed and each area was marked 1-5 with 5 being excellent. One area was 'local factors'. Jeffery had trained in Leeds Medical School, and we were expected to give 5 marks for 'local factors' to any applicant trained in Leeds. I was often paired for interviewing with a consultant gastroenterologist, Jean Wharton. Like me, she trained at the London Hospital many years before me. We rebelled. We gave 1 to anyone who trained in Leeds and 5 to anyone from anywhere else.

Training practices knew when they were not going to be allocated a trainee from the scheme and so had to advertise in the journals. It was difficult to make an advert attractive for someone to choose Castleford rather than Leeds, York, or the spa town of Harrogate. One could head the advert with 'Near the beautiful Yorkshire Dales'. The practice then had been to interview and select from any applicants. We never failed to appoint a trainee by this method.

The term 'trainee' was changed to 'general practice registrar' and then back to 'trainee'. Since 2007, these doctors are known as general practice specialty training registrars and course organisers, training programme directors.

It is always a good sign when a trainee is taken on as a partner by the practice where their training had been undertaken. My first six-month trainee was Anne Godridge, and I have described how we took her on as a partner in Chapter 8. She is now the senior partner. My last trainee was Deborah Hewitt. She became a partner at Tieve Tara. She always asked some of the most searching questions. Mostly these addressed her learning needs and made me think very hard. We visited a patient together who had been in the Royal Air Force. He had the typical handlebar moustache. Debbie asked me why some RAF men had moustaches like that. There is a Handlebar Club based in London that was founded in 1947. Members have to sport an appropriate moustache. I never properly discovered the answer to her question. My partner Anne Godridge became a trainer and two of her trainees became partners—Rosario Vega and Ben Young.

How are trainees assessed and certified fit to be a GP?

In the early years, a certificate was issued at the end of the training period that simply stated that the doctor had completed the training. There was no statement of competence until 1990. In 1996, summative assessment was introduced. Knowledge, solving problems, project work, consulting skills, and attitude were all assessed formally. Since I retired from general practice, a curriculum has been introduced and linked to the MRCGP, which is the single assessment.

Consultation skills were assessed by submitting videos of consultations. One could choose which consultations to include. Because of that it was really very strange if someone submitted a poor consultation. Was that poor insight or a poor trainer? I became a first-level video assessor. This work took hours and I did this at home. To fail someone was a very serious thing and there was an appeal process. The first-level failures were passed on to a pair of second-level assessors. These two assessors had to discuss the videos and come to an agreed conclusion. I eventually became a second-level assessor. I was rather soft with my assessments. My fellow second-level assessor was David Fyfe. He was tough, and I nicknamed him 'Fail 'em, Fyfe'. I actually think we made a good pairing. The videoing had to be uninterrupted by phone calls or someone knocking on the consulting room door. This was very difficult.

Trainers had to submit videos of tutorials in order to be reassessed. The same non interruption rule applied to these.

I decided to video a tutorial with Bert Van den Ende for my reassessment as a trainer. I used the study in my private house so all would be quiet. Halfway through, there was a knock on the door. It was another trainee, Paco Fernandez, who had come to ask me something. I could not believe it. As our house was semi-detached with the surgery, he had walked around, rung the doorbell, and Kath had shown him to my study.

Alison Evans was a research and development fellow at Leeds University, where she established, with the Leicester Deanery, a method of assessment of consultation skills using a simulated patient. The simulator had to learn a role and make it real for the trainee. This method was introduced as an alternative to videos in 2000. The feature that was so useful with this method was that the simulated patient could feed back how the consultation felt. The roles and the simulators were carefully chosen. The simulators were not actors. Over the years, I got to know two of them very well. One was a practice secretary and the other a social worker. The practice secretary, Karen Roberts, went on to manage the Yorkshire simulators.

A simulator was invited to one of our trainers' workshops, and we had the opportunity to feel what it was like to undertake a consultation. My 'patient' had a bald patch on his head. I decided to be naughty and pretended to be irritated and tired at the end of a long day. Was I being a simulated doctor? At the consultation progressed, the patient told me about the stress he was under such that I felt guilty about how I had started. I apologised and continued in an empathic mode. It became very real. The simulated patient gave me a very good feedback.

Failing the consultation skills element of summative assessment was very serious and generally resulted in that trainee undertaking a further six months of training. Failing on the second attempt usually ended their general practice career. This was very rare.

Problem solving was assessed by submitting a medical audit. I had become very interested in medical audit ever since Jeffrey Ellis asked me to teach on it at a trainee half-day release afternoon. I became a member of the Medical Audit Advisory Group of the health authority. This involved visiting general practices to try and encourage them to undertake medical audit. Medical audit should result in improving patient care. Let me explain medical audit with an example. It might be decided to undertake an audit of the taking of blood sugars in diabetics. A decision would be made that 90 per cent of diabetics should have an annual blood test for sugar. The first stage of the audit is to look at each diabetic and see what percentage had had this done. Let us say the answer came out at 70 per cent. A change would then be introduced in order to achieve the 90 per cent target. That might be that a letter is written to all of those who had not had a blood test inviting them to see a nurse. After a suitable time, the diabetics are looked at again and the percentage recalculated. The target of 90 per cent might have been achieved. If not, another change should be introduced and the cycle repeated. This is a simple description of a basic medical audit.

Alison Evans developed an alternative to the audit for trainees for this element of their assessment. A variety of types of project could be undertaken and submitted. This method was approved to be used nationally in 2000. It was called the National Project Marking Schedule (NPMS). The type of project could be a research study, a literature review, a clinical case study, a questionnaire, and so on. The submission was marked, using a schedule, by three first-level markers. If one or more of these felt the project was not up to standard, it was referred to two second-level assessors who had to agree. The second-level assessors might decide to invite the trainee to rewrite the project. If the resubmission failed, it was referred to national markers who were directors of deaneries. Most of the Yorkshire trainees undertook these projects, but nearly all trainees in the rest of the UK chose to submit an audit. The Yorkshire NPMS assessors were used to mark projects submitted from trainees in the rest of the UK.

The trainer had an opportunity to closely observe a trainee's work during the six months' attachment. At the end of the attachment, the trainer wrote a detailed report, which commented on attitudes as well as knowledge.

One method of assessing knowledge and attitudes was the Observer Structured Clinical Examination (OSCE). Trainees spent ten minutes or so at a 'station'. At a station, there might be a trainer with a task such as interpreting some test results, taking a blood pressure, or undertaking a consultation with one of us. After the time had expired, the trainee was moved to the next station. I manned a station with one of our receptionists, Hazel Bird. I had made up a role for her as a simulated patient. One of the trainees, Joy Issac, shone out. He passed our station with flying colours. After he completed his training, he worked in our practice for a short while as a locum. He became a partner in a practice in Castleford and is my GP at the time of writing.

When the OSCE was being explained to us trainers, my friend Grahame Smith said he thought the stations meant it was something to do with railways.

With my last trainee, Debbie Hewitt, I tested a personal assessment tool I had thought of. Of course, with each trainee I had the thought, 'Would I go to this doctor with my own medical problems?' Occasionally, the answer was 'definitely not'. My assessment tool was to take a real medical problem to the trainee and see how it was dealt with. I was overweight and at that time was not taking enough exercise. I asked Debbie to address the exercise problem. She was excellent, and we decided swimming might be the answer. After I retired as a GP, I joined a gymnasium and swim almost every day. I would certainly be happy to have Debbie as my GP.

The training, education, and assessment of both trainees and trainers are rigorous and have been of the highest standard in Yorkshire for the past thirty years.

Jean Lewis, a fellow trainer, persuaded me to consider applying for the post of GP tutor for the Pontefract district. In 1992, my application was accepted. This again involved an interview at the deanery in Leeds University. The job involved two afternoons of working at Pontefract Postgraduate Centre. It involved my approving applications for accreditation of educational events for GPs held in practices or other venues. A practice might invite a consultant to give a talk to the clinical team and that would require accreditation. Accreditation should ensure a good quality of the educational event. At that time, GPs had to undertake thirty hours of accredited education each year, and there had to be a balance between clinical, administrative, and other areas. Of course, a GP could turn up to an accredited educational event and pay no attention. It was rare for accreditation applications to be turned down. When I started, I had excellent advice from Elsie Green, the postgraduate centre administrator. She taught me how to fill in applications for the events I was facilitating. There were regular lunchtime lectures in the postgraduate centre. The teachers were mainly consultants. GPs were invited to these. The pharmaceutical companies sponsored most of the educational events. The sponsorship mainly took the form of providing food. There were evening events held in hotels, golf clubs, and other venues, and the drug companies would pay speakers' fees and any room charge. The drug company would try and persuade the GPs to prescribe their products. Sometimes a pharmaceutical company would try to hijack the meeting in order to strongly advertise their drugs. This was not allowed. A system of monitors was set up, and everyone knew that a monitor or I could turn up to an event uninvited. I once did this for an evening meeting held at the Darrington Golf Club. The speakers were Graham Hunter, a consultant gynaecologist, and Colin White, a physician, both of whom I knew quite well. When I walked in, I heard Colin say 'My God. It's him'. The drug company had brought the slides. I did not want to destroy my professional relationship with the consultants so I left them to it.

I tried to be creative with the educational events that I facilitated. I put on a series of lunchtime events called 'A day in the Life of . . .'. I would invite such people as the chief executive of the health authority or the hospice doctor to give a lecture.

We put on training session on how to improve consulting skills.

There was a session for GPs on drug misusers. This was the only training event where the health authority funded an attendance fee. The Wakefield District desperately needed GPs who would work with addicts.

We had a series of joint meetings for GPs and consultants on how to improve teaching skills.

I was particularly interested in multidisciplinary learning. We had a joint meeting for priests and GPs on spiritual care. I planned this meeting with the chaplain of Pinderfields hospital, Rev Roger Cressey. I got to know him well. A couple of years later, he helped me put on a huge event for which the speaker was David Jenkins, the outspoken former bishop of Durham. I invited anyone who worked for the NHS in the Pontefract district. We hired Pontefract town hall to accommodate the huge numbers of attendees. At that time, the administrative staff at the postgraduate centre had grown to three. Christine Sanderson had taken over from Elsie. She had Moira Fearnley and Pamela Wood to help her with this event. Christine was a superb manager of the centre and eventually became a practice manager in Normanton. The evening was sponsored by six drug companies and there was a packed house. Bishop Jenkins lived up to his nationally famous reputation as a firebrand. I remember his scolding us for not speaking out or doing anything if we felt the NHS was not performing at its best.

Another multidisciplinary meeting I put on was one for veterinary surgeons and GPs. I asked the hospice doctor to give a short talk against euthanasia. This certainly provoked discussion as vets use euthanasia extensively. One GP suggested vets should be used for euthanasia of

NHS patients! There was a vet there who was an expert on bereavement. A fellow GP confessed that he did not have a photograph of his wife in his consulting room but rather one of their late cat.

I was rather keen on debates. We again had to hire Pontefract town hall for a packed debate on fundholding. I have mentioned earlier how the introduction of this system divided the medical profession. It was a great debate, and the anti-fundholders won.

Before the general election in 1997, I invited each of the prospective parliamentary candidates for Pontefract and Castleford to a panel discussion on health. I had a rule that each candidate was allowed to bring only one guest. There were four prospective parliamentary candidates, from the conservative, liberal democrat, referendum, and labour parties. The first three brought their election agent as a guest. The labour party candidate, Yvette Cooper, brought an ex-miner from Knottingley who wore his flat cap throughout the meeting. Whatever question was asked about health, the referendum party candidate swung his answer so it involved an anti-Europe point. Labour was promising to abolish fundholding. This was one of the rare educational meetings that was attended by the chief executive of the health authority, Keith Salisbury. He was seriously told off by Yvette Cooper for not attracting more people to consultation meetings he had organised.

One of the most rewarding aspects of being a GP tutor was attending regular two-night residential seminars at the short course centre in Ripon. All the Yorkshire GP tutors got together for an exchange of ideas and to learn more about educational methods. Some of them had been GP tutors longer than me. I was made very welcome and over the following years developed a close working relationship with these colleagues. We were all very different. John Bibby burned the midnight oil poring over his practice's fundholding finances. Mark Napper went to bed early to get a rare decent night's sleep. He had three very young children.

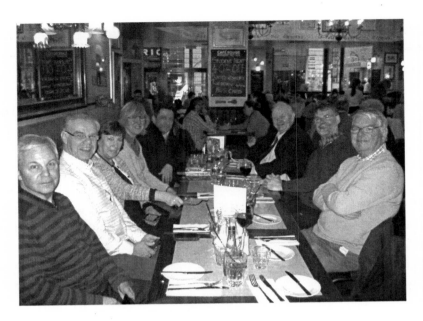

**Ex GP tutors at reunion in 2012. From left to right:
Martin Islip, John Bibby, Julia Taylor, Anne Parkin,
Sanjeev Kapur, David Ryland, John Moroney, and I.**

We packed as much as possible into the time at the seminar, and we continued working for a short while after the excellent dinner that was served with good wines. In the short course centre's lounge area, there was a fridge with alcoholic and other drinks. There was a book in which one signed for any drinks taken. For many years, I signed 'Jamie Bahrami'—the director's name. I was never charged for these drinks, and I did not know whether Jamie or the deanery paid for them. There was always a residential seminar before Christmas, and we had a special dinner at which Jamie Bahrami gave each one of us a bottle of port wrapped in Christmas paper. One Christmas, at Ripon, one of the GP tutors, Mike Scatchard, drank nearly the whole of his bottle before the end of the meal. We then went off to our favourite pub (The One Eyed Rat). Mike's legs gave him slight coordination and gait problems when we walked back to the short course centre. In later years, the course organisers joined us as participants of the seminars.

Jamie had four deputy directors—Andrew Belton, Alan Crouch, Brian Ormston, and Phillip Nolan. Each one of them contributed to the seminars to a greater or lesser extent. They also undertook inspections to practices, that had applied to be approved or reapproved for training. They undertook annual appraisals of the GP tutors and course organisers. During my time, working for the deanery, Philip Nolan appraised me seven years running. I got to know him pretty well and he was a great support. He was an expert in Neuro-Linguistic Programming and spent one afternoon familiarising us with this discipline. This was a method of communication that linked the brain, language, and behaviour. I found it a very difficult concept to grasp. To demonstrate one aspect, he asked for a volunteer. David Ryland stepped forward. He had had a serious argument with his practice manager. He was asked to sit on a chair with an empty chair in front of him. David was to imagine his practice manager was sitting in front of him and to say something to her. Philip hoped David could solve the problem by having a conversation with his imagined practice manager. David refused to do this on the grounds they weren't speaking to one another.

In 1996, I applied to be a course organiser at the Pontefract Postgraduate Centre. I did this for two years and was at the same time a GP tutor. The only other person at that time who had done both jobs was Alison Evans (the research fellow in the department of primary care at Leeds University). I joined David Brown at Pontefract Postgraduate Centre. He had taken over as course organiser from Jeffrey Ellis.

I found the job of course organiser difficult and challenging and was grateful that David was so good at it. We had to organise the half-day release programmes for trainees and the workshops for trainers. The first half-day release session for trainees that I facilitated was like a trade union meeting. The main topic they wanted to talk about was payments for undertaking extra work (overtime) in their hospital training jobs. I felt out of my depth. Trainers generally taught on the half-day release afternoons and the course organisers dealt with administrative matters. We had the difficult task of meeting consultants to look into reports of poor teaching. GPs involved with training experienced a lot more learning about educational methods than consultants. One of the most complex tasks was working out three-year job plans for the trainees. The three years had six half-year attachments, four of which were in hospital training posts and two in general practice. David was expert at sorting all this. I spent a lot of time trying to set up a system such that the trainees spent their two six-month GP attachments in contrasting practices. It must be good to work first in a practice in a deprived area with the second attachment being in an affluent area. Another interesting experience would be to work in a small practice and then in a large one. I never got this off the ground. I was a course organiser for only two years. One interesting course organiser appointment at Pontefract was Susan Butler, who was not a trainer. She argued that the job was one of organisation not teaching. It was the first time a non-trainer had been appointed as a course organiser. Jamie Bahrami was creative in the appointments he made. He appointed two GP tutors with nursing backgrounds—Julia Taylor and Jan Firth. I was not really suited to being a course organiser. I have GP tutor's blood coursing my veins.

Towards the end of the 1990s, Pontefract Vocational Scheme merged with Wakefield and Dewsbury to form the West Riding General Practice Education Centre. Half-day release teaching rotated around each site and the course organisers worked closely together.

In 1999, Alison Evans had a new Leeds University course approved. This was the postgraduate certificate in primary care education. It was a two-year part-time course and it was offered to all the GP tutors and course organisers. It was a third of a master's degree. Most of the GP tutors and course organisers took up her offer to undertake this course. It was hard work with assignments to write and be marked as well as attending for regular afternoons of teaching. Some of the GP tutor/course organiser seminars were devoted to the certificate work. I did a lot of the assignment writing early in the morning before going to work. One of the assignments was on the analysis of an organisation of our choice. I chose the Castleford Choral Society. David Brown chose

Merry Maids, a domestic cleaning company he uses for his house. There was another assignment on curriculum development and one on adult learning. The final module was a choice of either mentoring or research. Two others and I chose research and the remaining twenty or so the easier area of mentoring. Our tutor for the research module was Alison Evans, who was high powered and taught me a lot. I was proud to be awarded the certificate. This qualification gave the course organisers and GP tutors significant street credibility when it came to planning postgraduate GP education.

Michael Peake, a consultant chest physician, was the hospital's education tutor. We worked together closely. In the early days, Jean Lewis, Jeffrey Ellis, Mick Peak, and I would invite one another and our partners for Sunday lunch or an evening meal. Mick left to undertake a job in Leicester. His job was taken over by a consultant rheumatologist, Andrew Harvey. We shared a very small office in the postgraduate centre and often worked there together, which was rather cosy.

Another of Jamie's ideas was to develop a mentoring scheme for GPs. In 1996, my fellow GP tutor at Pinderfields Postgraduate Centre, Mark Napper, and I were asked to pilot the training of a group of GPs as mentors. The training sessions were generally in the evenings and were facilitated by Derek Powell, a senior consultant from the training organisation International Training Services Ltd. Funding was from the Yorkshire Deanery. Recruitment was difficult. There was virtually no response from a letter to each GP. We decided to headhunt GPs we knew to have good listening and empathetic skills. These were telephoned, and we started with a group of seventeen. Mark and I were members of the group and undertook the training. The initial aims were to encourage personal development, reflection, and provide support for the mentees. The training involved studying videos of our mentoring one another. My co-mentor for this was Liz Moulton. A couple of years after this training, she mentored me through a very difficult partnership problem. We developed a close working relationship over subsequent years. The training was repeated at all the postgraduate centres managed by the Yorkshire Deanery, and this resulted in about 100 GPs becoming mentors. My first mentee was a GP who had had a complaint from a patient. We met in my house and the meetings could last well over two hours. Mentors did not receive any payments for this work. Since the training, I have mentored GPs, a nurse, PCT staff, and most recently a consultant. Two important mentoring skills are listening and being non-directive. Mentoring has been a most rewarding experience and led me to work with helping ill and underperforming GPs. One of the trained mentors, Jeremy Belk, wrote to me telling me how good the training on the pilot had been and that he was giving up general practice to become a full-time counsellor.

Trainees were encouraged to attend a residential summer school. These were at the Ripon site at first and later at York University. The summer school involved we tutors living there for four nights. The short course centres had bedrooms for the tutors and as the training college students were on holiday, their rooms could be used for the GP trainees. Hotels in Ripon were also used. The trainees spent the whole of the daytime in a sub-school of their choice. The choice of sub-school included management, consulting skills, and ethics. I was asked by Jean Lewis to join her, Bill Message (a solicitor, and Jean's partner), and Ron Mullroy (the course organiser at Wakefield) as a tutor on the ethics sub-school. The course was run by Brendan Carroll. We had pre-course tutor meetings over dinner at Jean and Bill's house. We were joined at one of the meetings by Prof. Tim de Dombal, a consultant gastroenterologist from Leeds, who was an expert in medical ethics. I learnt such a lot from being a tutor on that course. Tim gave a fascinating lecture on how it is impossible for doctors to know everything. He told us that in the past year there were 8,000 papers published on gastroenterology alone. We looked at such things as confidentiality, the abortion act, how to judge something as ethical, creating autonomy, the paternalistic approach, and so on. At the end of the day, we usually debriefed outdoors so Ron could have a cigarette. We also held tutorials outside if the weather was good.

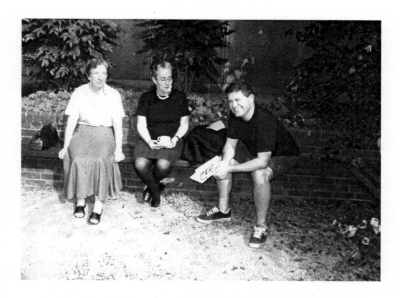

**Alison Evans, Maggie Eisner, and Mark Purvis,
tutors at a York Summer School.**

After dinner, there would be master classes for both tutors and trainees. Every year there was an organ recital performed by Geoffrey Coffin. He was one-time assistant organist at York Minster and had restored many organs including the one at the summer school. I also spent time relaxing by playing one of the pianos in the music department. After three years of teaching on the ethics sub-school, there was a coup. I am not sure who staged the coup. We were not asked again and the ethics course was then managed by Stuart Calder. Stuart ran a wine tasting master class. He had a rather unique skill. After he had tasted a wine, he could project it from his mouth into a spittoon that was situated about five yards away. I was involved with another summer school later in my career, which I describe in the next chapter.

Over the years, I was tutor for three medical student attachments. I found introducing medical students to general practice more difficult than trainees partly because the former were not allowed to prescribe. The student would do a consultation alone and then I would go to their room and spend five minutes going through things and issuing a prescription if necessary. I would be doing a surgery at the same time as the student and had to make sure I ran exactly to time. I was also expected to assess the student. Certainly with my last student, the assessment was taken into account when allocating house officer jobs. I found this quite a responsibility.

John Lee was my first student and he became a partner.

The second was James Mair, the son of my close friend Geoff who was at medical school with me. Geoff died in 2002, eighteen months after a heart—lung transplant to cure a complex lung problem. James was a chip off the old block and he lived with us for the two weeks of his attachment. He was at St Mary's Hospital, London. He particularly enjoyed a teaching session I had set up with our undertaker, Trevor Morritt. I had been on this session with a trainee and knew it was of good value. Trevor first told him what his job was about and how GPs had to examine bodies after death if there was to be a cremation. This was to eliminate foul play and check on the cause of death. They then went to Pontefract crematorium. There they saw the ovens and had an explanation of how bodies were dealt with as well as their ashes. James is now a successful GP in Norfolk.

My third medical student was Jenny Goodenough from St Thomas's Hospital, London. She is the daughter of Alan and Marie, friends since my youth. She was most conscientious, had a flashy sports car, and thoroughly let her hair down at one of our practice parties. Unfortunately, she did not see the light and become a GP. She is well on the way to becoming a plastic surgeon, and I am sure she will own a Porsche in the fullness of time.

In 2002, I spent a couple of years as a clinical educator to our district nurse, Jackie Spencer. She was undertaking an M.Sc. course that would qualify her to be a nurse practitioner. It was a relatively new concept to have nurse practitioners in primary care.

The course was based at Huddersfield University and was created and run by Prof. John Lord. John was at the same time a practising GP and a fellow GP tutor.

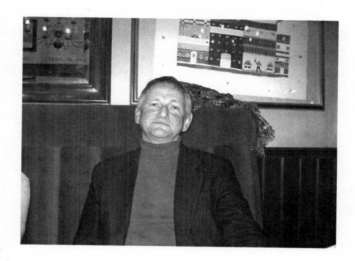

Prof. John Lord in 2012.

I had always worked very well with Jackie and I found this education work fascinating. I found one scholarly paper that showed that patients would rather have a consultation with a nurse than a GP. I think I realised why this was so when I started tutorials with Jackie. She was intrinsically kind and frequently gave the patient a reassuring touch. She also addressed most of them with the northern 'luv'. There was a very detailed curriculum and many checklists for us to complete as part of the assessment of her competency. You can see from Chapter 4 (Clinical Medical Student) what she had to be taught and learn. She had to be competent at taking a history, examining a patient making a provisional diagnosis. A nurse practitioner would be consulting unsupervised and allowed to prescribe a limited list of drugs.

A male doctor should always have a chaperone in the consulting room when undertaking an intimate examination of a female patient. This could be a female relative but more often one of the practice nurses or receptionists. It was an interesting experience for me when Jackie asked me to be her chaperone while she examined a man's testicles. She had assignments to write and attended Huddersfield University. This was as well as continuing with her job and looking after her family. She was successful in achieving the M.Sc. after submitting a 10,000-word assignment on drug misuse. Our practice decided that we did not want to employ a nurse practitioner so Jackie moved to a neighbouring practice to start her new career as a nurse practitioner. She works mainly with patients with mental health problems.

From 1994 to 2000, I was the vice chairman of the Yorkshire Postgraduate General Practice Education committee having been the GP tutor representative. It was Jamie's idea for me to have that post, and I began to realise what a force he was in my medical journey. He is my third educational hero. (The first two were J. Z. Young and Bill Keatinge).

This was a big committee whose members included the deputy directors, the professor of primary care, course organiser representatives, and so on. I was extremely anxious when asked to chair the meeting in the absence of Keith England, the chairman. I had read a book entitled *The Chairman's Guide*. I thought this covered everything. The book even gave advice as to when to call the police if a meeting got seriously out of hand. I was convinced I had thought of every possible event. After about twenty minutes into the meeting, scrabbling and scratching noises were heard coming from above a false ceiling. Then a pigeon flew out. I had to suspend the meeting. Jamie Bahrami climbed on a table and opened a window and we eventually got the bird to fly out. That event was not covered in the notebook. Fortunately, during the period of suspension of the meeting, no motions were passed!

In 2000, I started a new phase of my career. I resigned as GP tutor and course organiser and took up a post of associate director of postgraduate general practice education at the Yorkshire Deanery. I continued as a trainer until 2002.

CHAPTER 10

THE YORKSHIRE DEANERY

Jamie Bahrami, the director of postgraduate general practice education, had hinted to me that if I applied for the new post of associate director of postgraduate general practice education, there was a very good chance of my being appointed.

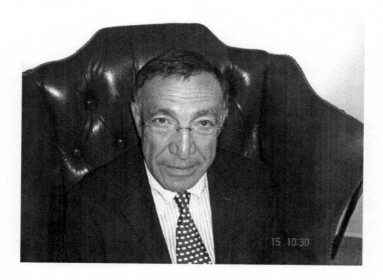

Jamie Bahrami.

The job involved working four sessions a week. A session was about three and a half hours or half a day. The interview at Leeds University involved my making a ten-minute presentation to the panel. The interviewing panel was daunting. The chairman was George MacDonald Ross, a philosopher who was an expert on Liebnitz. The others included George Taylor, deputy director of the department of general practice at Newcastle University; Alison Evans, whom I wrote about in Chapter 9; Jamie; and Rosemary MacDonald, the Yorkshire dean of Postgraduate Medical Education. There were two applicants. One had travelled from New Zealand and was interviewed first. When I was called in, I was so nervous that I was breathless from hyperventilating.

After my presentation, each of the interviewers was invited to ask me questions. When it got to Jamie, he said, 'I know Richard well enough. No questions'. I was offered the job before I left the building. Rosemary MacDonald told me that the first applicant had presented far too many slides. She liked my slide of the quotation of J. Z. Young from his book *Doubt and Certainty in Science* (see in Chapter 3) so much that she asked for a copy. I was over the moon.

The deanery building was situated on the Leeds University campus. One of Jamie's deputies, Philip Nolan, showed me around the deanery and the University of Leeds campus. He told me a dry route he used to get to a cafe on a rainy morning where one could enjoy a hearty fried breakfast.

I was the first associate director to be appointed and that was in 2000. Soon after, further such posts were advertised. Adrian Dunbar, Mark Purvis, and Alison Evans joined me. Mark and Adrian were course organisers. We worked in a small office where each of us had a desk, computer, telephone, and space for storage and files. Alison was a great support. She was an innovator and researcher. Mark arrived at work very early and started the day with loud music filling the office. Adrian is a proficient athlete and cyclist. He would often arrive on his bike and enter the office wearing a Lycra suit.

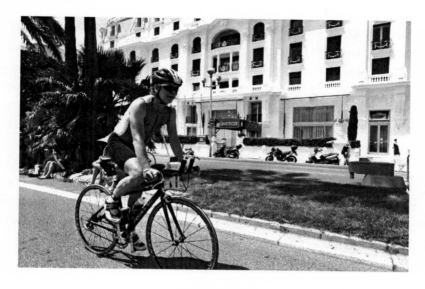

Adrian Dunbar.

Jamie's office was down the corridor, and if his door was open, one could go in and discuss anything. Jamie and I met regularly to plan my work.

The role of the deanery included overseeing the education and training of all the doctors, including hospital doctors, and dentists in most of Yorkshire. South Yorkshire was covered by another deanery. The population of the whole of Yorkshire is between five and six millions. South Yorkshire has a population of about 1.3 million. The population that the Yorkshire Deanery covered was double that of Wales and similar to that of Denmark. There were thousands of doctors registered and working in Yorkshire and a similar number of dentists.

Each associate director had areas of responsibility. Jamie asked me to manage the National Project Marking Schedule (NPMS). This method of assessment of trainees' project work was described in the last chapter. Our deanery managed the marking of submissions from the whole of the UK. Like the assessment of videos of consultations, we had first—and second-level assessors. There were also national assessors, and these were six of the directors of postgraduate general practice education. Jamie Bahrami was a national assessor. I was a second-level assessor and that helped me feel what it was like to be a marker. The three first-level assessors did not communicate and were unaware of one another's marks. If there was a failure at first level, the project was referred to second level. The project could be a choice of a questionnaire, a notes review, a literature review, a case study, research, the planning of a new service in the practice, an audit, or a discussion paper. Processing payments for marking was undertaken by Barbara Innes, who also set up meetings and marker training sessions. This was a big job for her.

The competencies assessed were the ability to make a logical argument, communicate it in English, as well as the ability to plan and sustain an activity over a period of time. The second-level assessors had to agree their marking and a discussion usually took place over the phone. It was evidence of her dedication to work that I discussed one project with my fellow second-level assessor, Alison Evans, while she was in her bath at home. As part of my final module in the postgraduate certificate, I wrote a literature review. I gave it to Jamie to mark as if it was a submission for the NPMS. To my horror, I only just passed. It was a very serious problem if the second-level assessors agreed to fail a submission. Any such failures were sent to two national assessors who made the final decision together. The national assessors were directors of deaneries. Each year I sent them projects to mark to assess their competencies.

My job was to make sure that the skills of the assessors were maintained at a level such that the system was quality assured and therefore fit for purpose. I therefore ran regular training sessions (calibration) for our markers throughout the year. We had to recruit new markers as more and more submissions were coming from outside Yorkshire.

I could not have done all this work without the help of a senior administrator at the deanery, Claire Conlon. Indeed, when I started, I think Jamie asked her to be my minder. Claire also collated all the marks.

I undertook familiarisation and training sessions for potential markers in other deaneries. I visited Oxford, Maidstone, and Barnsley. I ran one national in Leeds for the whole of the UK. The most memorable visit was to the North of Scotland Deanery. I was invited by Rowland Spencer-Jones to a hotel in Nairn and I stayed for three nights. I decided to travel by train. It was a wonderful experience travelling the eight hours from York to Inverness in a first-class seat. Castleford to Nairn is just less than 400 miles. It was the North of Scotland Deanery's trainers' workshop. At the start of my session, huge map of Scotland was represented on the floor of the room. Each trainer made an introduction and then stood on the map where he or she worked. They had come many miles from places like the islands of Mull and Skye as well as other remote places. Unlike our trainers' workshops in Yorkshire, these colleagues could meet only a couple of times a year at a hotel. The expense for the deanery must have been huge. I felt a great responsibility to deliver a high-quality session. They made me most welcome. I enjoyed the evening meal where the conversation included a discussion as to how to deal with a deer that had been shot. One GP from a small island had only a few hearty patients to look after. He was also the island's warden for the Royal Society for the Preservation of Birds. One perk for me was that I was taught to appreciate Laphroaig single malt whisky. It is pronounced 'la-froyg' and means 'the beautiful hollow by the broad bay'. At the end, I was presented with a bottle of malt whisky as a thank-you present.

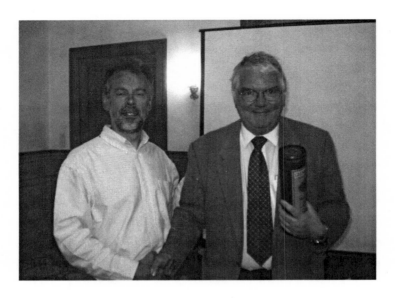

Rowland Spencer-Jones and me, Nairn.

A few months later, Rowland phoned me and reminded me that I had not quite finished all the teaching. He invited me to return. I travelled by air the second time to do another session of training.

The formal assessment of trainees was summative assessment. One could not practice as a GP without passing summative assessment. Jamie asked whether I could take his place as an observer member of the National Summative Assessment Board. I was to regularly report to them on the progress of the NPMS. The board's members were very senior GP educators and mostly directors of deaneries. It was chaired by Steve Field (West Midlands dean) and later, Agnes McKnight (Northern Ireland director). The board was responsible for overseeing the various elements of summative assessment. These were the assessment of consultation skills by either video or the simulated patient, the assessment of written work by either the audit or NPMS, the assessment of knowledge by multiple choice questions, and the structured trainer's report.

My membership of this committee introduced me to high-level medical politics for which my mentor and tactical adviser was Jamie Bahrami. I was also lucky to be working with Alison Evans, who developed the NPMS. Most trainees in the UK chose or were persuaded to submit a COGPED audit rather than a project to be marked by the NMPS. COGPED is the Committee of General Practice Education Directors. It was COGPED that approved that particular audit method as an assessment tool. The audit tool was developed by Prof. Stuart Murray and Dr Murray Loch from the West of Scotland Deanery, both of whom were members of the National Summative Assessment Board. Yorkshire's method of assessing written work, the NPMS, was resented by most of the committee. I felt very alone in fighting for our marking schedule. I knew we had several directors of deaneries behind us because of invitations to familiarisation sessions and submissions of projects. I was continuously being asked to prove our method was as good as the COGPED audit. I was asked to send a batch of projects with the marks to Prof. Dame Lesley Southgate, the then president of the Royal College of General Practitioners. She was to study them and comment on our method of marking. Back at the deanery, I spent hours collating and comparing marks and calibrating the markers. I truly believed in our method of marking as did the West of Scotland in theirs.

Going to the meetings of the Board was a big expense for our deanery. I travelled to the meetings by first-class rail because I did not want to leave early to catch a specific second-class train. For afternoon meetings, I could travel there and back in one day. I was once summoned to a meeting that was held in a very smart hotel in South Gloucestershire. There was no convenient railway station so I travelled by car. My wife came with me, and we stayed in a hotel in Birmingham. I was at the meeting for only twenty minutes. This was my last meeting and I did say, 'I wish that someone would tell me "Richard. You have done a good job. Thank you"'. No one said a word. However, Professor Murray wrote some nice words to me when I left the deanery. The West of Scotland won the battle hands down. In about 2005, the NPMS and the Leicester method of assessing consultation skills were dropped.

The approved methods of assessing these two areas were the West of Scotland's audit and video. Chapter 12 describes how trainees are assessed in 2012.

When I was seeking to be a trainer, I attended the 'O' course, described in Chapter 9. This course was replaced by two mandatory seminars for prospective trainers, introductory seminars 1 and 2. Jamie's deputy, Brian Ormston, managed the training and assessment of prospective trainers and asked me to join him as a tutor on seminar 1. Brian taught me such a lot on that seminar. He has been a great support and advisor to me while I was at the deanery.

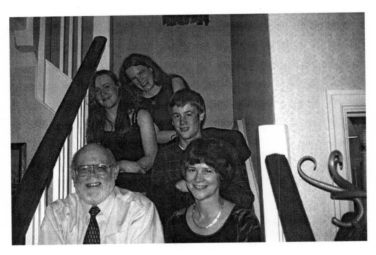

Brian Ormston and some prospective trainers.

However, he continued Martin Rogers' tradition of everyone having to learn one another's name. This time he allowed us to make notes. Even so, when it came to my turn, I was so anxious again that I could not remember the name of a GP who worked in my area and whom I knew really well. One of the main features of the new seminars was that the prospective trainer had to bring videos of his or her consultations. It had been established that a GP who is not good at consulting will make a poor trainer. Our fellow tutor on that seminar was Roger Higson, a course organiser working from Masham in the Yorkshire Dales.

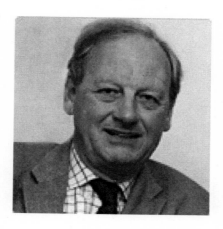

Roger Higson.

There were no more than twenty-four attendees on the seminar as more than eight in a small group is not good educationally. Commenting on videos in a group resulted in learning about giving constructive feedback. We practised tutorials. They were taught about summative assessment. Of course, my area for this was the NPMS. The prospective trainer had to undertake more preparatory work to bring to seminar 2. After a while, Brian asked me to run seminar 2, and I was joined by course organisers and trainers Liz Moulton (my mentor) and Elaine Powley. This seminar took place twice a year.

Elaine and Roger ran a seminar for GPs on the relationship of the arts to medical education. This was a fantastic seminar, and one GP from my area told me that it had been the best seminar he had ever attended. Elaine did a session one evening on our seminar 2. She read from a novel about a death. There were tears in our eyes. It taught us that fiction has a lot to teach us about human life. 'Fiction is a window on to the world—a mirror of human behaviour and experience—and it may give penetrating insights into human feelings and emotions.' This is a quote from Roger and Elaine's book.[20]

---

[20] Elaine Powley and Roger Higson. 2005. *The Arts in Medical Education. A Practical Guide*. Radcliffe Publishing Ltd. p. 30.

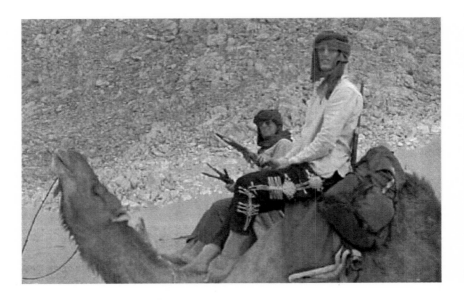

Elaine Powley on one of her exotic holidays.

Liz Moulton was a very skilled educator with a completely different style of teaching from me. She was particularly good at doing things spontaneously, which has the advantage that identified learning needs could be addressed there and then. I prepared in advance in detail, like I did when I was a lecturer in physiology. Liz was an expert, among other things, in teaching consultation skills. One idea of hers, which was fun, was for the doctor to role-play the worst start of a consultation that he or she could think of. There was one I will never forget. The patient entered the consulting room to find the doctor injecting into a vein in his arm.

After attending the two seminars and a positive assessment by the tutors, applicants were invited to a deanery interview. The format of the interviews at the deanery changed over the years so as to be not so daunting. There were usually no more than four interviewers, one of which was Jamie. Either I or the chairman of the Postgraduate GP Education Committee ran these interviews. It was a surreal experience for me when I chaired the interview of my partner and first full-time trainee, Anne Godridge. Jamie was in a somewhat playful mood, and I had to tell him to behave himself. Anne was approved as a trainer. This was greatly to her credit and the culmination of several years of effort on her part. Not only did she give birth twice during that time but also passed the MRCGP.

Liz Moulton asked me to join her at the trainees' summer school. She ran a course for the trainees on consultation and counselling skills. The first one I was involved with was at Ripon. However, Ripon was eventually bought by a private company, and we moved to York University. The other tutors were Maggie Eisner and Bryce Taylor. Maggie was an expert on social class issues, ethnic differences, and dealing with diversity. She taught so well how GPs should consult and recognise their own prejudices that may influence rapport and empathy. She was the course organiser for the Bradford vocational training scheme. Later in her career, she wrote medical reports on people who had been tortured.

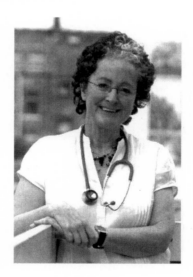

Maggie Eisner.

Bryce Taylor was a national expert in counselling and helping people. He worked for the Oasis School of Human Relations. He has written several books and was a close friend and colleague of Liz.

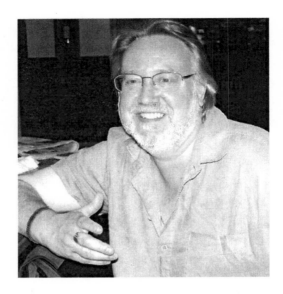

Bryce Taylor.

Let me describe two examples of his work that he brought to the summer school.

There was a session about dealing with patients' problems. The group (about twenty-four trainees) was to be divided into smaller groups of three (trios). Each was to think of a problem and on a scale of 1-10, it should be about level 3. In the trios, one would be the GP and he or she would discuss the second member of the trio's problem. The third would be an observer. At the end of a fixed time, each would give feedback. Each person would take a turn at each role. The strength of this method of learning was that the 'doctor' would get feedback not only from the 'patient', but also from an observer who was not intricately involved with the 'consultation'. To start the ball rolling, we did a demonstration to the whole group. I thought of a problem and Bryce was the GP or helper. The problem I thought of was one I had with my hairdresser. I thought this was at level 3 of seriousness. However, Bryce brought out of me all sorts of complex doctor—patient relationship issues such that towards the end of this demonstration, I felt it was at level 8. The trainees were great about this. One even found out there was a barber on the campus and suggested I got my hair cut that afternoon so I did not have to go to the hairdresser for a long time.

On 28 February 2001, Jamie was on his way by train to a meeting in London. The train crashed near Selby and he was very seriously injured, having to be transported to a hospital in Hull by an RAF Sea King helicopter. Ten men died in that accident, and the driver was later jailed for five years. We were all devastated about this news. He made a slow but sure recovery over the following months, and Brian took over as acting director.

At the 2001 summer school in Ripon, which was held in September, I had had my breakfast and was on the way to our main teaching room. I passed a clutch of people glued to a television. They were watching footage of the first aeroplane crashing into one of the twin towers on 9/11. Of course we were all shocked to the core. There were a couple of Muslims in our group. One was particularly upset as she felt Muslims would be blamed for many years to come. We suspended our plans and Bryce facilitated a session so we could deal with our emotions about this tragedy. There were tears. I found out later in the day that Brian Ormston's daughter was on an underground train in New York at the time of the event. She was uninjured.

Bryce died suddenly at the relatively young age of 63 in 2010. His book *Working with Others, Helping, Counselling and Human Relations* is one of my bibles.[21] In it, he states that the core conditions of effective helping are genuineness, empathy, and warmth. These are developed and discussed in detail. These core skills can be used in counselling, consulting, appraising, mentoring, and friendship. It was a great privilege for the trainees to spend nearly a whole week learning with Bryce.

---

[21] Bryce Taylor. 1998. *Working with Others. Helping, Counselling and Human Relations*. Oasis Publications.

Liz Moulton's book *The Naked Consultation*[22] is based on a handbook written for GP principals and nurse practitioners to improve their consultation skills. In Chapter 3, she states 'good beginnings make good consultations'. However, there is a cautionary note: 'Sometimes changing the way you begin consultations has unexpected consequences. One of my colleagues, a distinguished and popular local doctor, tried beginning his consultations in silence, after going on a course. He was rewarded by a succession of patients who were completely thrown by this behaviour, which was very different from normal, and asked him instead whether he was, in fact, ill today!'. Anyone reading that would not realise that the doctor was me!

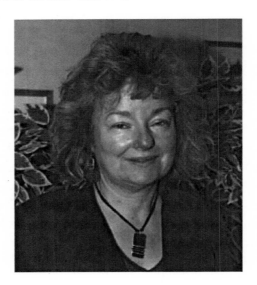

Liz Moulton.

After Jamie returned to work and we planned the retraining and reaccreditation of the Yorkshire GP mentors. There were about 100 of them. Janice McMillan was a senior educationalist working for the deanery. She had had significant experience with mentoring. We undertook the training together. The training took a number of months as the two-hour sessions could accommodate only sixteen

---

22   Liz Moulton. 2007. *The Naked Consultation*. Radcliffe Publishing.

GPs at a time. One aspect of the training was to use simulators. Their roles were GPs with problems. I looked up the literature and no one had used simulated doctors before. One of the roles was a GP who was getting depressed about his work and had an alcohol dependency problem. The simulator made sure a shoelace was undone and his tie was not straight. He also dabbed a little whisky on to one lapel of his jacket so the mentor could smell alcohol. The simulators were fantastic and provided powerful training. I found it fascinating writing the roles and seeing the simulators develop them.

The core work of each associate director included appraising course organisers and GP tutors. The geographical area covered by the Yorkshire Deanery was divided up between us. We also organised the GP tutor/course organiser seminars. We dealt with trainees who had failed summative assessment. This involved visiting his or her postgraduate centre and meeting the trainers and course organisers involved. A decision had to be made whether to fund any retraining. This was a very big decision as one cannot have a career as a GP without passing summative assessment.

On a couple of occasions, I went with Jamie and others to a student hall of residence in Leeds to meet fourth-year medical students. The objective was to persuade them to become GPs. The first time we did this was a very pleasant experience. After some presentations, we each facilitated a discussion with a small group of students. We went again a couple of years later. The atmosphere had completely changed. It was an unpleasant experience in that a significant number of students believed that general practice was boring and academically beneath them. These views could have only come from their consultant teachers. There was always a cultural gap between hospital doctors and GPs. This was an evidence of how the gap was created. We never went again.

We were shocked when Jamie Bahrami told us of his intention to retire. I think the train crash was a significant factor in his decision. He and his wife sold their house in the UK and moved to Spain, where they are very happy. George Taylor from Newcastle was appointed as our next director. He was on the interviewing panel for my associate director's post.

In the time between Jamie's announcement and George's arrival, there was a GP tutor/course organiser's seminar that I was very much involved with. I gave a presentation at the start of the seminar. It was a PowerPoint presentation entirely of pictures and set to music. I did not utter a word but changed the slides at appropriate times. One was a photo of Jamie accompanied by 'The leader of the pack' by the Shangri-Las. That pop song faded into the start of the first movement Haydn's Surprise Symphony. On hearing the very loud chord (the surprise chord), the screen went blank, and there was a period of total silence both from the music of the presentation and from the audience. The silence was ended by fading in a photo of George Taylor accompanied by more music. One of my colleagues, Paul Robinson, told me later that this was truly poignant. It was meant to be.

Just after Jamie left, I was thrilled to hear that colleagues had nominated me to become a Fellow of the Royal College of General Practitioners. The person who had most input to this was Alison Evans. Kath and I had a lovely two nights in London. Bill and Anna Bullingham came from Cheltenham with their daughter (and my goddaughter, Rachael). They treated us to a celebratory dinner the evening before the ceremony. It cost a one off payment of £700 to become a Fellow. Each new male fellow is given two ties, one green and the other blue. These can be worn only by fellows. As I walked out of the room where the ties were being distributed, a colleague remarked to me: 'those are the most expensive pair of ties I have ever bought'. Five of us from the Yorkshire Deanery became Fellows that day. The four in the photograph knew one another well.

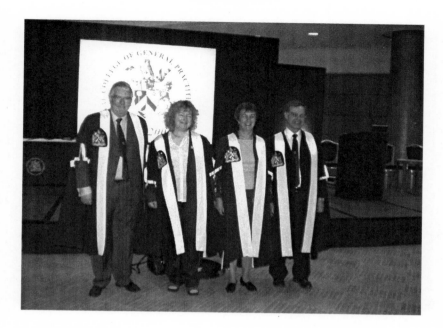

FRCGP 2002. From left to right: Me, Liz Moulton, Shelagh Bullimore, and John Bibby.

I felt somewhat lost after Jamie left. In 2004, I had heard there was a job about to be advertised for a GP adviser, protected learning at the Eastern Wakefield Primary Care Trust (PCT). The headquarters were based in my home town of Castleford. I had an informal meeting with one of the directors of the trust, Gill Galdins. She persuaded me to apply and I was offered three sessions, which I accepted. I handed in my resignation at the deanery shortly after Liz Moulton was appointed as an associate director. This was not exactly tactful timing. My colleagues gave me a great leaving dinner and some wonderful presents. It was time for a final career move.

CHAPTER 11

THE PRIMARY CARE TRUST (PCT)

I had entered yet another world. The Eastern Wakefield PCT was responsible for managing opticians, dentists, pharmacists, nursing homes, and so on. The PCT's geographical area included Castleford, Pontefract, Hemsworth, Ackworth, Featherstone, and other small towns and villages. Although GPs are mostly self-employed, practices have a contract with the NHS. The PCT was involved in agreeing and monitoring these contracts. It commissioned (planned and paid for) health services provided by Pontefract Hospital. It also provided community paediatricians, health visitors, and district nurses. There were many other activities performed by the PCT. The PCT directly employed managers, administrators, and secretaries. The PCT had a budget of many millions of pounds. Its headquarters was in the old Castleford and Normanton District Hospital. My office was a converted lavatory. The office area in that part of the building was very cold in the winter. Sometimes staff had to go home early because of the cold. The electricity system was so old that extra heaters could not be used. After several years of this discomfort, I decided to complain. As an expert in hypothermia, I thought I might have some authority. I wrote to the chief executive. I recorded some room temperatures. I pointed out that I believed that the organisation was breaking the law (the Factories Act). I also wrote that the only way I could see of keeping warm was to have office sex. The very next day work was started to improve the situation by installing double glazing, and so on.

My job involved facilitating large educational events for primary care staff. These were held at Pontefract race course. These took place several times a year during an afternoon. These were for GPs. Nurses, primary care staff, and practice managers mostly had separate educational events organised by us. Sometimes they all learnt together. All of these educational events took place on the same afternoon. It was a major organisational task. Anthony (Tony) Nicholas, the PCT's events manager, was responsible for the management of these events. I worked closely with him and tried to ensure a high quality of education.

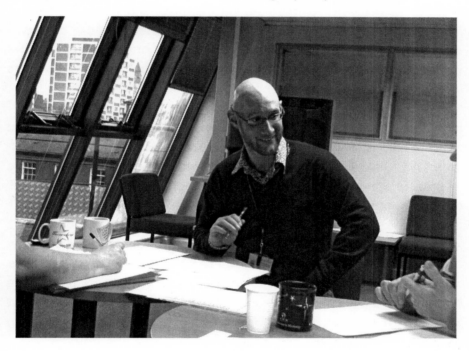

Tony Nicholas.

On up to ten afternoons a year, the vast majority of practices closed down for education. They undertook no clinical work. The out-of-hours deputising service dealt with any medical problems. On four or five of those afternoons, education took place in the GPs' surgeries or at a venue of their choice. The remaining afternoons were used for the large educational events described above. This education system was called TARGET (Time for Audit, Research, Guidelines, Education, and Training). This method of primary care education was the brainchild of Dr Martyn Coleman and others from Doncaster. TARGET had been taken up by most of the country's PCTs. Our sister PCT, Western Wakefield, ran similar events, but these were managed by their medical director, Dr Mark Napper. Mark, like me and most of my GP tutor colleagues, had moved to work for a PCT.

After a provided lunch, the large educational events started with a keynote lecture. Prior to the meeting, delegates chose two workshops from a choice of up to seven. After the lecture, they attended their two workshops separated by a break for tea. Four or five administrators were drafted in from the PCT to help on the day. The number of teachers involved in a TARGET event in the racecourse was significant.

How did we decide what to teach? Tony sent out a questionnaire to all GPs, nurses, and GP administration staff towards the end of each year. This asked for their learning needs as well as what the balance of outside and in-house education should be. We also had a TARGET development committee that included some GPs and a nurse. The PCT also had ideas as to what should be covered. Hospital consultants were keen to tell primary health-care workers about their services and how these should be used. Both Tony and I had to prioritise these requests. Sometimes we allowed a consultant to have a ten minute slot at the beginning of a big event. Sending out the survey to GPs had one great advantage. It was not uncommon for one of them to say to me 'Who decided to teach on this load of rubbish?' My reply was 'You did'.

A lot of doctors think that they are born with teaching skills. There were sometimes seriously boring presentations where PowerPoint slides had only black-and-white typed bullet-pointed phrases that were read out in a monotone. As time went on, I had the courage to point out to some consultants what made a good presentation. I might have risked being labelled as cheeky when I requested one or two consultants to be creative. I was pleased that my requests were often taken up.

I tried to make the education have an element of fun. After the merger, we asked Dr Nadim Nayyar, a Castleford GP, to introduce and chair the big TARGET meetings. He has a fabulous sense of humour. He was employed by pharmaceutical companies to chair meetings and has made several TV appearances. His introductory remarks, sometimes risqué, were usually sent to me prior to the meeting and I acted as his censor.

One of the most popular keynote lectures was by Martin Davies, whose background was in psychiatry. He was also a well-published cartoonist. He had us all crying with laughter. His talk was about doctors looking after themselves. After a significant time into his presentation, he showed us a cartoon of a miserable woman. He told us he had drawn it earlier and that it was of one of the women GPs, entering the building. He then said, 'And she still looks like that now'. Of course, the cartoon was fictional.

We never got to grips with what education was going on in practices when they closed down for an afternoon. Generally, my own practice might have an education meeting possibly followed by a partner's business meeting. I was quite relaxed about what the GPs in other surgeries did on those afternoons as they would welcome some time to reflect and catch up on paperwork. However, auditors of the PCT's finances might not have been so happy with this relaxed approach should they have discovered it.

It is important to evaluate educational events. There was an evaluation form to complete at the end of the event the results of which Tony collated and sent out to the teachers. If an event was to be repeated and there was a problem with the evaluation of a workshop or lecture, then this could be addressed before the second session. Of more use was a late evaluation. One of my fellow GP tutors, Martin Islip, had had success with these for GPs in Leeds. He produced, with the help of other GP tutors, a booklet in 2003 called 'Development without

Tears'. In that booklet is an excellent explanation of evaluation. We wanted to find out whether the teaching session could result in better patient care. Late evaluation response rates are notoriously poor. However, we had a reasonable response which was mostly positive and encouraging.

The planning of each these big events was perfected to a fine art by the events manager, Tony. If he got the right people together, we had just one planning meeting and the rest could be done by email. I usually went with Tony to this first meeting.

In 2005, I decided that Tony was such a good events manager that we could put on a national conference in Wakefield. The event was to be the Fifth National Protected Learning Time (PLT) conference. We persuaded the PCT to underwrite any losses. I put forward my idea at a meeting of the National Association of Primary Care Educators who offered to plan the content. Maive Lamb, from Northern Ireland, was a major contributor to the planning. The keynote first presentation was from Martyn Coleman, who, as I mentioned earlier, pioneered TARGET. The conference was a success, and we three wrote it up in the main GP Education journal, *Education for Primary Care*.[23] The conference generated a significant profit for the PCT, which we put in our education account.

The PCT director responsible for this part of my work was Helen Mortimer. She was most supportive and left us to get on with our work. Helen knew I had worked for the Local Medical Committee's professional support group, looking after and assessing ill and underperforming GPs. She asked me to take on this support and mentoring role for the PCT. This took significant time but the work was intermittent. Any disciplinary action was decided at director level together with the chairman of The Professional Executive Committee, Dr Phillip Earnshaw, a GP. There were very few GPs for whom the

---

[23] Sloan, R, Nicholas, A and Lambe, M. 2006. *Fifth National Protected Learning Time (PLT) Conference: A Valuable Resource or a Waste of Time? Education for Primary Care*. 17, pp. 506-10.

PCT had serious concerns. However, was this the tip of an iceberg? Could there be another Harold Shipman?

Harold Shipman was a GP who worked in Todmorden, West Yorkshire. He was a serial killer of his patients and was convicted of fifteen murders in January 2000. He hanged himself in Wakefield prison in 2004. He was highly regarded and was suspected only when another GP noticed the high death rate in his practice. (He worked for a while as a junior doctor in my local hospital, Pontefract. There was a letter from him to my mother in the records of one of my patients.)

I had to visit practices that had reported a concern about a partner, see GPs in their homes, meet GPs regularly in my office, and deal with the National Patient Safety Agency. The agency has a role to prevent and manage performance problems. I was involved with the agency in developing and monitoring a performance plan for a GP. Some of the GPs we tried to help retired, others were suspended by the PCT, and a very small number were struck off the register of the General Medical Council.

A couple of months after starting working with TARGET, one of the directors, Gill Galdins, asked me to add a fourth session of work for the PCT. She asked me to manage the GP appraisal scheme. I accepted her offer. I took this management role over from Susan Moloney, who was head of human resources. I think she was greatly relieved to hand over as it had been significant additional work for her.

The first thing I did was to set up a training and familiarisation day to recruit some new appraisers. I undertook that course myself and became one of the appraisers.

As a result of the course, two or three appraisers joined the group of originally appointed GP appraisers. Julia Taylor, the GP tutor, was facilitating the support work for the appraisers. I joined her with this work until she retired. The administration of the appraisal scheme at the PCT was undertaken by first Pauline Kenny and later, Janine Heptinstall.

Appraisal was introduced for consultants in 2001 and for GPs the following year. The appraisal scheme for the Eastern Wakefield PCT had been operating for a couple of years before I started working there. It is mandatory for a GP to undertake an annual appraisal. For the appraisee, this involved collecting evidence of training, audits, meetings and significant events. These were then written up on a template either on the Internet (The NHS Appraisal Toolkit) or in a typed document. Sometimes the document was handwritten. This information was made available to the appraiser a few days before an arranged meeting. The meeting was usually at the appraisee's surgery and could last up to three hours. As an appraiser, I found it fascinating to look at a fellow GP's work in such depth. Over the six years I was undertaking appraisals, I met some really outstanding doctors. I am sure patients did not fully appreciate the amazing skills and expertise of most GPs.

The appraisal interview looked at last year's personal development plan (PDP) to see whether objectives had been achieved. The appraisal process was a formative one. It was not, therefore, a serious problem if an objective in the PDP had not been achieved. That objective might be discarded or put into next years' plan.

There were GPs with special interests (GPwSIs). They were experts in fields such as dermatology and musculoskeletal problems. These GPs had had very significant postgraduate education in these areas and ran outpatient clinics in the local hospital. It might be that their learning and development was biased towards their specialty rather than general practice. I never found that any of these GPs neglected their general professional development. I appraised GPs with large medical business interests. These interests included ownership of companies that bought up practices and walk-in centres. Part of the appraisal was to look at possible probity issues. For example, is there a conflict of interest for a GP who is married to a pharmaceutical company representative? What about the GP who part owns a pharmacy? There were GPs married to consultants. I explored whether these GPs ever referred patients to be seen privately by their spouses. Another part of the process was to look at relationships with colleagues. This was where partnership and staff problems and worries were discussed and some of these were significant. The relationship between GPs and their consultant colleagues changed over the last fifteen years I was working in that they hardly met face to face. Communication between GPs and consultants was mainly in writing. The appraisal interview usually ended with the drafting of a PDP. The plan might include intended courses, undertaking an audit, or maintenance. Maintenance means keeping up to date generally. This is a huge task for a GP. One method of addressing learning needs was to keep a learning diary. Every time a learning need was identified, it could be entered into the diary and looked up at a later time. There was software available for computerised learning diaries.

After the appraisal interview, the appraiser wrote a report. This could be done on the Internet on the appraisal toolkit. At first, GPs were reluctant to use the Internet. In 2002/3 only three used the toolkit. One of those was myself and I gave up halfway through because I found it too complicated. As appraisal lead, I tried to encourage the use of the toolkit and in 2009/10, 238 out of 240 GPs used it.

The final stage of the appraisal process was for each to sign it off as a true record. In 2010, appraisers were paid £540 for each appraisal. I thought that was a lot of money but others did not. It upset Janine and Pauline, who were processing the appraisals, when an appraiser wrote a poor report and was being paid such a lot. I totally agreed with them and indeed stopped sending two appraisers any more work.

In 2007, the Eastern Wakefield PCT merged with its Western counterpart. There were some redundancies including our chief executive, Mike Grady. I was very sad about his leaving as he was a great motivator and knew his people well. My area of responsibility doubled without any increase in our team. The merging of the TARGET education systems was managed like clockwork by Tony.

The merged appraisal schemes resulted in there being seventeen or so appraisers covering about 250 GPs and locum GPs. The Western Wakefield PCT appraisal scheme was managed by the medical director, Mark Napper. I took over his work and became responsible to him. The enlarged scheme was administered by Mark's personal assistant, Jenny Miller. She was one of the most efficient administrators I had ever encountered.

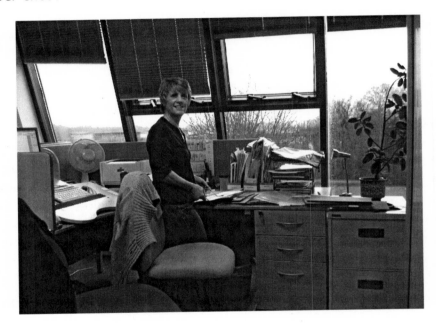

Jenny Miller.

I decided to re-interview the appraisers after advertising to all GPs in the Wakefield District. After the interviews, contracts were issued.

At the start of the merged scheme, the GPs were asked to choose their appraiser. There were two or three very popular appraisers who undertook a large number of appraisals. I undertook about twenty a year. We never solved the problem of the GPs wanting their appraisal at the end of the appraisal year, that is, February and March. This resulted in a huge workload and was very difficult for those appraisers who were also full-time GPs. After three years with the same appraiser, the GPs were asked to change. This was to try and prevent collusion.

I had appraisals as a GP, a trainer, GP tutor, course organiser, associate director, and with my job at the PCT. Grahame Smith, my friend and GP, was my first appraiser for my GP work. Some might say this was too cosy a relationship that would foster collusion. However, he had a truly professional approach with me and helped me with my professional development. One of the most important appraisals was my last one as a GP, knowing I would be retiring from that work. Janice Woodrow spent nearly three hours with me in the appraisal interview. She pointed out that I would always be a doctor even though I was no longer helping patients.

In 2008 (I had retired as a GP), I persuaded the PCT to allow and fund Liz Moulton to undertake my PCT appraisal. She knew me well and was the deputy director of Postgraduate General Practice for the Yorkshire and Humber Deanery at that time. I was her GP appraiser for three years. She has often said 'the most important part of appraisal is praise'. Readers may be surprised to learn how rare it is for a GP to be thanked or praised for all their hard work.

I continued to run the monthly support group for the appraisers. This was held at lunchtime in Wakefield. The two groups of appraisers had to get to know one another with the merger of the PCTs. After an ice-breaker, we usually discussed any problems the appraisers might have. The problems were sometimes quite worrying. There was a locum GP who hardly ever read anything medical and his appraiser could not see how that doctor could possibly keep up to date. Was that person dangerous? I wrote and asked to see that GP but never received a reply. I reported this to Mark Napper, my director, who sorted it out. There were GPs who did not engage with the appraiser and thought the appraisal was a waste of time. They submitted very little paperwork.

There were GPs who repeatedly failed to fix an appointment with their appraiser and others who only produced the paperwork at the appraisal interview. These problems were possibly a reflection of the GPs' approach to their work.

At the support group meeting, I always tried to get us working at improving our appraisal and reporting skills.

I played an interesting trick on the appraisers on one occasion. I brought an appraisal report I had written about a locum I had supposedly recently appraised. The report was actually entirely fictional up but I did not tell them that until the very end. The report indicated that the locum was fed up with his work and possibly depressed. I had to role-play my feelings and answer questions. At the same time, my written report was of a mediocre standard. They were learning how to do sensitive and positive feedback to me. They needed this skill when feeding back to their GP appraisees. It is difficult to repeatedly facilitate creative learning events.

I found that in the last two or three years, I was devoting three of my four sessions to appraisal and one to TARGET. It was the other way round at the start. This was partly because there was an annual report to write as well as an annual quality assurance process to undertake. Every year I read the appraisal documentation for each of the 250 or so GPs and extracted salient points. Once a year I had a one-to-one meeting with each appraiser and fed back my opinion on the quality of their work. I must admit that when I met Martin Lannon, we spent about fifteen minutes discussing his work and the rest of the time talking about the humorous articles he writes.

Another reason for my increased workload was the Labour government's proposal to introduce revalidation. Dame Janet Smith was asked by the government to undertake an inquiry into the activities of Harold Shipman with an obvious objective—preventing such murders ever happening again. Her first report came out in 2002, but it was the fifth report of 2004 that made significant comments and recommendations about the appraisal scheme. The report stated, 'Evidence recorded by the Inquiry suggested that appraisal for GPs was purely a formative process, not capable of providing an evaluation as to fitness to practise.

'. . . the standards to which it was being carried out were variable. If appraisal is intended to be a clinical governance tool it must be toughened up.'

We all thought that Harold Shipman would get through the appraisal process without anyone suspecting he had any problems. He was a popular and well-liked GP. It was a GP from a neighbouring practice, Dr Linda Reynolds, along with Deborah Massey, a local funeral director, who reported the Shipman practice's high death rates to the coroner.

Revalidation would involve every five years, evidence from a more robust annual appraisal as well as other information examined by a responsible officer and a decision made as to whether that doctor is fit to practise. The responsible officer was to be Mark Napper.

To prepare our appraisers and GPs for revalidation, I first became a member of a Leeds-based West Yorkshire revalidation group of appraisal leads. This later was subsumed by a revalidation support group covering most of Yorkshire. We met in Sheffield at Amar Rughani's surgery. Andy Godden, GP tutor, Sheffield, facilitated these meetings. These two colleagues were deeply involved with the Royal College of General Practitioners' development of revalidation. They were very experienced educationalists and have published widely. Most of my former GP tutor colleagues had, like me, moved to jobs working for their PCT. It was good to meet up with John Bibby (Bradford and Airedale PCT) and John Moroney (North Yorkshire and York) again. It was a privilege to be a member of that group. There were huge variations in both the finances and the management structures of the different PCT's appraisal schemes that had to be ironed out before revalidation was introduced.

The date when revalidation would start was put off year after year. I therefore continued with our appraisal scheme as it was. I retired from the PCT in May 2010 and still revalidation had not been introduced. It will start in a small way in 2012.

The PCT asked me to be involved with a team of people who would travel to Madrid for a long weekend in order to recruit Spanish doctors to work in the Wakefield and Leeds areas as GPs. This was a nationally funded project. It is cheaper to do this than to educate a medical student and then train a doctor to be a GP. The team consisted of me, Wendy Pearson (a director of our PCT), George Taylor (director of postgraduate general practice education, Yorkshire), Dr Damian Riley (from Leeds PCT), and a lecturer from the Bradford Language School. We had to assess about twenty applicants and the three doctors worked as a team assessing their medical knowledge, skills, and attitudes. Their language and communication skills were also assessed in detail. In the end, we selected six. Three were to go to Leeds and three with us. Before a final decision was made, they came over for a couple of days, and we showed them the practices that had volunteered to employ them as salaried partners for a year. The salary of GPs in Spain is significantly less than that in the UK. We arrived at a two-man general practice and I pointed out the partners' cars. One was a Porsche and the other a Jaguar! After completing a huge amount of paperwork, they were allowed to settle in the UK and work as a GP. My friend and colleague Grahame Smith and I facilitated a six-month induction course. The three working in the Wakefield area were Gonzalo Galaza, Paula Alba-Mendez, and Jorge Esclapez. These doctors were truly excellent and most conscientious. They put some of we UK GPs to shame. (I was lucky to work with a Spaniard, Rosario Vega, whom we took on as a salaried partner at Tieve Tara. Like the others, she was an outstanding GP). The government funded their practice salaries for the first year. Jorge returned to Spain. Paula is Gozalo's partner. They bought a house and are now happily settled and working as locums.

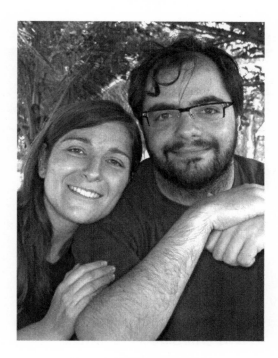

Paula and Gonzalo.

The Quality Outcome Framework (QOF) was launched in 2004, and I described the impact of this on our practice in Chapter 8. I decided to become a QOF medical assessor. I was able to undertake this work in addition to appraisals, PCT, and GP work because I had dropped down to three days a week working in my practice. I retired from the practice in 2005 and spent the next five years with plenty of time to accommodate QOF assessments.

The QOF was managed at that time by Fiona Nash. She dealt with all the applications for the job of QOF medical assessor. The new QOF medical assessors had to have significant training. We went in a group to the Queens Hotel in Leeds for the first of two training days. Facilitators came up from London from the Department of Health. Our group from Wakefield was admonished for being too light-hearted and laughing too much. There was role play. One domain of the QOF was about blood pressures and hypertension. Blood pressure targets were set for hypertensive patients on treatment. For one role play, I was the assessor and the scenario included my suspicion that the GP was cheating and falsifying blood pressure readings to achieve the target. Dr David Brown undertook the role of the GP. I tried as best I could to delicately approach the problem. David, taken aback, said, 'Are you accusing me of fraud?' This shocked me somewhat, and I dealt with it in my own way that was probably not very good. However, I entered into the spirit and said, 'I would like to move on to the second area of suspected fraud, please.' There was a lot to learn about the huge number of targets that covered not only clinical areas and disease but also administrative areas such as record keeping and education and training.

I was on holiday for the second day of training in Leeds. I travelled the 218 miles to Weston-Super-Mare for that. My wife, Kath, came with me, and we stayed in a hotel on the way back home. These national training days must have cost the NHS a fortune.

Each year since 2004, the QOF has been evolving with some targets being removed and new ones added. In 2010/11, the QOF had four domains—clinical care, organisational, patient experience, and additional services. My role as a medical assessor was to look at and check the results for the clinical care domain. This had eighty-six indicators (targets) across twenty clinical areas such as coronary heart disease, asthma, depression, and dementia. The NHS Information Centre (http://www.qof.ic.nhs.uk) is a web site where one can access an individual general practice's QOF results. It also explains QOF in some detail.

In the Eastern Wakefield PCT, QOF inspections were undertaken by a team of three. There was a medical assessor, a PCT manager, and a layperson. The layperson usually looked at the patient experience and staff areas. I particularly enjoyed working with the lay assessors Brian Dunderdale and Bill Clift both of whom I knew for many years outside of my medical world. The PCT manager usually looked at the organisational domains. A practice manager became part of the team round about 2008.

At the start of each QOF year (1 April to 31 March), all of the assessors met to decide which domains and indicators to inspect. It was impossible to inspect them all. There was one area we chose where most practices were having some difficulty.

Before each inspection, there was a significant amount of paperwork to read and analyse. This could take a couple of hours.

The inspection took about up to three hours. After introductions with the practice team, I went off with a GP to a computer. I chose patients at random in order to inspect the relevant indicators to see whether targets had been attained. This process was supposed to be confidential. There was a complex computer programme that could anonymise records, but this was rarely used. One GP had cut out some cardboard to cover up the patients' details on the computer screen, but soon after we started he discarded it. Over a six-year period of my inspections, confidentiality did not worry most practices. I did not recognise a single patient I was ever shown. One practice was somewhat obsessed with confidentiality and postponed the inspection twice at the last moment. This was because the computer programme to anonymised records was not working properly. Eventually I did my inspection there with a colleague who was also my friend. When we had finished, he asked whether he could discuss a case with me. He put up the patient's records, and the name and address were fully displayed! On another inspection, I was working with one GP at the computer in his consulting room. A second GP sat on the examination couch. Each time a patient was put up on the computer, the second GP said, 'Do you know Mrs Thing or Mr So-and-so?' I did not recognise any of them. In the end, for fun, I replied, 'Yes, she is my second cousin'. The GP on the couch was Andrew Sykes, who had been a trainee of mine years previously and was then (and is at the time of writing) the chairman of our Local Medical Committee.

One or two practices provided us with a generous buffet lunch, but others never even offered us a cup of coffee or tea. I was called 'dear' for the first time in twenty-five years by a woman partner when she asked whether I wanted anything to drink. Was this some form of mild bribery?

Before leaving, we met with the practice team and each of the inspectors fed back our findings. We always praised the achievements, and I hope gave helpful advice on how to achieve targets in the time remaining of the QOF year. On occasions there was a negative reaction from the practice and sometimes this was followed up by writing about the perceived problem to the PCT.

I wrote up the findings at home and emailed them in to the QOF manager. These were then collated with the findings of the other two inspectors and a report put together and sent to us to check. That report was then sent out to the practice with a copy to the chief executive of the PCT.

Fiona Nash, who managed the QOF, left to work in Doncaster. Her job was taken over by Kevin Duggan.

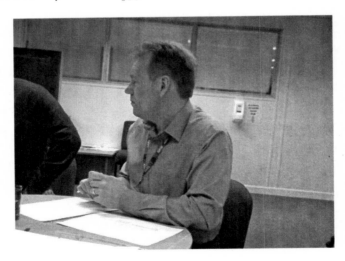

Kevin Duggan.

Managing QOF for forty or more practices was a huge job. I worked in the same open plan office as Kevin and got to know him well. He discussed with me queries practices had. These queries were often trying to get around the rules. Over the years I have been amazed at what colleagues have come up with to legally bend the rules. The approach reminded me of what goes on with legal tax avoidance. I was asked to go to another PCT and do a quality assurance inspection there. One practice was seriously bending the rules. Fortunately, I was not involved in any decision as to what to do about this but simply had to give in my report.

In 2010, a medical QOF inspector was paid just over £900 for the work for one inspection. PCTs varied as to how much was paid and how the scheme was managed. However, one can calculate that the management of QOF by my PCT costs over £40,000 in medical assessor payments. PCT management salaries were also very significant.

The maximum number of points that could be attained in 2010/11 was 1000 and the payment for each point was £127.29. Achieving the maximum points earned a huge amount of money for the GPs. Of course there are expenses involved in managing and achieving targets in a general practice. This 2004 contract resulted in GPs throughout the UK receiving a massive increase in salaries, sometimes to over £100,000. Naturally, the GPs were determined to reach the targets and most attained very high points. However, in my opinion, achieving these targets has seen the most significant improvement in health and health care of a general practice population in the whole of my medical career.

In 2006, I decided to set up a group for retired GPs and locum GP. I called this the Educational Support Group for GPs without a Base (ESG). It sounds as if, to become a member, one has to have a particularly serious anatomical defect. Locum work can be a lonely business. The meetings were a way of the PCT thanking locums and GPs who had retired for all their hard work. I continued to run this group after I retired from the PCT and am still doing this at the time of writing. We meet monthly either at my ex-surgery or at a venue in Wakefield. We usually, but not always, have a guest. The meetings do not always have a medical theme. We have had talks from the chairman of the Wakefield Advanced Motorist's Association; on 'coping with the credit crunch'; Dr John Waring on the Rotary Club's campaign to eradicate polio in India; Dr Ruth Kent on neurological rehabilitation; Dr Philip Barker on astronomy; Dr Grahame Smith on clinical hypnosis. There have been arranged visits to our newly built Pontefract and Wakefield hospitals as well as one to Wakefield Prison. We had a tour in 2011 of some new eco houses that were being built near my house.

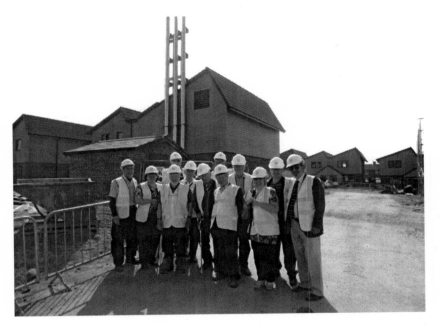

Some members of the ESG.

Dr Debika Minocha had a great idea that we brought newspaper cuttings about medical matters for the group to discuss. George Ward told us about freemasonry.

In 2009, I sent each member an evaluation questionnaire. There was an appreciation of maintaining contact with young and old. One doctor was encouraged to come out of retirement and to start work again. Networking was important. I asked them to suggest a new name for the group to replace our cumbersome one. One suggestion was the ROGs (Richard's Old Geysers). Another was the LADS (Learning for Ancient Doctors Society). We stuck to the ESG.

The colleagues I worked with and met at the PCT were hard working, creative, and conscientious. Improved patient care was always the motivator for them. When I retired in May 2010, we had a lovely lunch together so I could say goodbye and thank them.

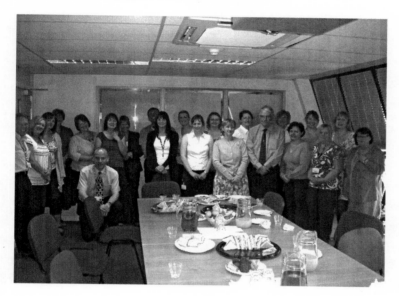

Colleagues at my final day at the PCT.

CHAPTER 12

2012

This chapter resulted from talking with people who are at a place in 2012 now that I visited on my journey, which spanned sixty years.

In Chapter 1, I described my middle-class upbringing in a medical family. My wife and I had no children and live in the house in which I was brought up in. Since the building of the new medical centre the house is completely separate from the surgery. The windows of the surgery that overlook our garden have been bricked up. We have a gardener and Maureen, aged eighty-seven, is our housekeeper since 1978. We have always used a driver when we go out in the evenings to friends, a restaurant, and so on. We have had two drivers over the years both of whom were patients. The first was Derek Turner and now is Kevin Tansley. I arrange the lifts with Kevin by email. When Kevin arrives to take us home, he texts me 'outside'. What a luxury! We had a second home in the Yorkshire Dales for twenty years and now have a house in Umbria, Italy. I know several GPs who have second homes. We are in that lucky generation who have had a good income, excellent pension arrangements, low mortgages, and benefited from a property boom. I know one or two families where the parents are doctors. One of my friends and colleagues Liz Moulton married Richard Lewis, who is a consultant cardiologist. They have three sons who went to the same school as me (Queen Elizabeth Grammar School, Wakefield). Two of the sons are pursuing a career in medicine and the other is a scientist. Liz maintains that it was the school (now private) that facilitated her sons' considerable academic successes. My second cousin Lorna married Stewart, and they are both GPs. They too have a house in Italy. The children of most GPs I know have done as well as I did at school and have been brought up in a middle-class atmosphere. The youngest GPs of today, like other young people, are struggling with the high mortgages required to buy their first home. They don't have housekeepers or gardeners, and they drive modest-sized cars. I think I had a more privileged upbringing than the children of the GPs of today.

Prof. Christopher Dean introduced me to Daniel Wornham, who was in his third year of an intercalated B.Sc. in his department of anatomy at UCL Medical School. University College Hospital merged with the Middlesex Hospital in 1987 to form the University College and Middlesex School of Medicine (UCMSM). In 1998, the Royal Free Hospital School of Medicine for Women merged with UCMSM to form the Royal Free and University College Medical School (RFUCMS). In 2008, it was renamed the UCL Medical School. This medical school is one of the largest in the UK and is often ranked in the top five.

The A-level requirements for entry to the MB BS programme there at are three grade As with one in biology and another in chemistry. In addition, there should be a pass in an AS level and preference is given to those who study a contrasting non-scientific AS subject such as history or geography. A statement is sent from the school. There is also a personal statement by the candidate. Dan had worked part-time as a health-care assistant in a hospital and loved that work. I am sure that counted for a lot in the decision to select him.

As well as the minimum A-level requirement, there is an entry examination. This is the Biomedical Admissions test (BMAT). As well as UCL, passing the BMAT is required to become a medical student at Oxford, Cambridge, the Royal Veterinary college, Imperial College, and the University of Bristol. This is a two-hour written paper with multiple choice and short answer questions as well as an essay. Most other medical schools require success at the UK Clinical Aptitude Test (UKCAT). This examines verbal, quantitative, and abstract reasoning as well as decision analysis. There is then an interview. Subject to passing these entry requirements, an offer is made. One then becomes one of the 350 new entry medical students. Each student undertakes a three-year B.Sc. degree before moving on to a clinical medical school.

The first two years of the degree are devoted to the study of the fundamentals of clinical science. Anatomy, biochemistry, physiology, and pharmacology are taught using a system of modules. Examples of these modules are Foundations of Health and Disease; Infection and Defence; Fluids, nutrition and metabolism; Cancer biology. There are lectures, demonstrations, practical classes, as well as dissection of a human body.

Professor Dean took me and Dan to the state-of-the-art dissecting room. Because of the huge number of students, the year is split into two for dissection. This means that a body is shared between two groups of about eight. The teachers include retired consultants who do that work voluntarily. I met Andrew Heaton, a retired A & E consultant. He trained at Guy's Hospital and told me that in his day one was allowed to smoke in the dissecting room to cover up any unwelcome odours. Some GPs who also teach and are paid a nominal fee. There was a great buzz of sound and activity. I was impressed by the relaxed and empathetic relationship Chris Dean had with the students. There were shelves on which were specimen jars, some of which were in the dissection room of my day. I met a technician, Laurence Clark. Part of his job was to look at the work done after a session and record dissection that was outstanding on a board.

Throughout the two years, there is a module called the Professional Development Spine. This involves students learning how to examine a patient and go on community and hospital ward placements. They are taught about evidence-based medicine and medical ethics.

At the end of each of the first two years, there are examinations. These consist of multiple choice, extended matching questions, multiple essays, as well as an objective structured practical examination. There is also a multiple choice exam looking at scenarios.

There is computer learning that can be accessed from home. There is online histology teaching.

The third year offers the chance to study subjects in more depth, look at research literature, and undertake a project. One or two students are allergic to research and can choose a library project. The work is divided into course units (cu) and to be awarded a degree with a class (first, second, etc.); four units must be completed and passed. Because of the size of UCL, there is a huge number of affiliated research supervisors and a very large choice of combinations of course units. Dan was undertaking his degree in anatomy and developmental biology. His courses are mechanism of development (0.5 cu), neurodegenerative disease (0.5 cu), cancer biology (0.5 cu), and an experimental laboratory project (1.5 cu). The first three courses involve an examination at the end of the year and perhaps a 1,000-word dissertation. Dan was researching the effect of a drug on osteoporosis by looking at its effect on osteoblasts. (Osteoblasts are cells that produce a substance that is the basis of bone). Osteoporosis is thinning of the bones partly because osteoblasts reduce in number with age. The osteoblasts were grown in Petri dishes. His supervisor was Tim Arnett, professor of mineralised tissue biology. For this work, he had a space in his supervisor's laboratory. The research course ends with a 9,000-word dissertation. Dan and his supervisor had just heard that an abstract had been accepted for a conference at which Dan will present their work.

The UCL Medical School aims that 90 per cent of the students will obtain either a first or upper second-class B.Sc. degree.

The curriculum for the six years is continuously developing and there changes will be made for the intake in the autumn of 2012.

After the iB.Sc., the 350 students will be allocated to one of three clinical teaching campuses—University College, The Royal Free, and the

Whittington. There they will study clinical medicine for the remaining three years.

I will leave it to readers to compare my experience of preclinical and the Anatomy B.Sc. with Dan's. I believe that the education I had at UCL from 1963 to 1966 was superb. That education has evolved so that all students experience a year with research and this must be a good thing. It would be interesting to find out how the research experience has impinged on those students who became GPs. I am disturbed by the high A-level grades required for entry now compared with my time. Should all doctors be so good at examinations?

One of my teachers had a building named after him.

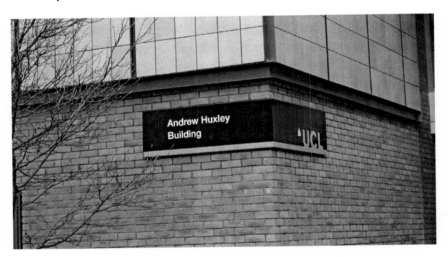

Building named after my professor of physiology

The lecture theatre where I heard J. Z. Young's first lecture to us is now named after him.

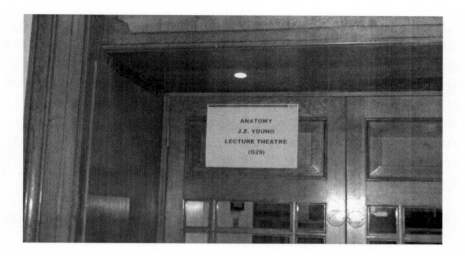

The J. Z. Young lecture theatre

One afternoon in May 2012, I met three junior doctors in the old London Hospital Medical College building. They told me about their clinical student training as well as what work was like as a foundation year-one doctor (FYI—the equivalent of a pre-registration house officer).

Emile Kahn is an FYI doctor who lives at home and wants to be a rheumatology consultant. Natasha Atchamah comes from the London area and is also in FYI and hopes to be a GP. Viyaasan Mahalingasivan is also a Londoner and FY2 doctor and intends to work in renal medicine. There is no longer hospital accommodation for FYI doctors and Natasha and Viyaasan live in rented properties. Although I kept my private rented accommodation on during my house jobs, we were provided with hospital accommodation both at Mile End and the London.

Seventy per cent of the intake already have a primary degree. There were about half a dozen students with degrees in our year.

At the beginning of the three-year clinical student course, there is a four-week introductory course. For most of the rest of the time, they work in firms. The firms could have many consultants, not just two like our firms. Because the student intake can be 400, these attachments can be not only in district general hospitals scattered in the greater London area but also in places like Colchester. Indeed none of Emile's firms were undertaken at the London Hospital. They agreed it was a good experience studying away from the London Hospital. The number of students on a firm could be one or up to ten. All do a firm of cardio/pulmonary medicine as well as a long attachment with a medical and then a surgical firm in the third year. Sometimes at the end of a firm, they might go out for dinner with the consultants.

Pathology is studied throughout and histopathology is computer based. Microscopes are not used.

There is a total of about five weeks spent in a general practice. There was no teaching on general practice in my day.

There is a brain and behaviour module where psychiatry is learnt. There is a locomotor module that covers rheumatology, dermatology, and orthopaedics. All the subjects I was taught are covered in the clinical course at Barts and the Royal London Medical School.

However, obstetrics and gynaecology training is very different. Because of the high number of Asian women in the East End of London, male students are not welcomed in the delivery room. The obstetric training involves observing and maybe helping at five deliveries. They also observe an abnormal delivery and a caesarean section. That there are 400 students in a year must make it impossible for each to deliver babies at a place where midwives are also being trained. Certainly in general practice, the midwives have taken over the GP's work with pregnant women, and it is possible that there is no longer a need for obstetric experience at the same level as was taught in the past.

There are no tutors outside of the firms but each has a supervisor for the three clinical study years. That supervisor is rarely seen and then only when there is a perceived problem.

I will describe the assessments that have to be passed to obtain the part 2 (second) MB BS (finals).

There is a continuous assessment throughout the three years of clinical training and this is part of the second MB BS examination (finals). At the end of each year, there are examinations. These test core knowledge and its application. Data interpretation is assessed. There are modified essay questions testing problem solving and there are extended matching questions. There is a computer-based assessment of 100 single best answers (multiple choices) with images and other materials. Communication is assessed at stations observed by an examiner. Simulated patients and manikins are used. The vast majority of students pass their final examinations and become FY1 doctors.

Before the first day practising as an FY1 doctor, there is a three-week 'Preparation for Practice' course. This involves shadowing the FY1 doctor whose job will be taken over. The ward sisters are still excellent resources for the steep learning curve there is at the start of the first FY1 job. Because of the European Work Directive, no more than forty-eight hours can be worked each week. (We often worked more than 100 hours a week as a house officer).

There is a basic salary plus extra (banding) for antisocial hours, and so on. Two or three different FY1 jobs are undertaken in that pre-registration year. They learn time management, prioritisation, and the management of the acutely ill patient. There could be thirty patients to look after on a ward.

The work of the A & E department is far removed from that of the receiving room in 1970. It is a tertiary-level accident centre. It dealt with multiple victims from the July 7 terrorist bombing and receives patients from multi-vehicle accidents. The only NHS air ambulance (helicopter) in London is based there and has a catchment out to the M25 motorway.

At night, I (a pre-registration house officer) and one nurse manned the receiving room. FY1 doctors are not allowed to work in the A & E department. At night, there might be two or three FY2 doctors, two registrars, and one or two consultants on duty.

There is no hierarchical behaviour in the A & E department. First names are used by everyone and it is a very friendly department. Jobs are undertaken by anyone depending on skills rather than seniority.

No one wears a white coat any more. We kept our stethoscope in one pocket of our white coat and the British National Formulary book in the other pocket. Today the stethoscope is worn around the neck.

Despite the modern doctor is working less hours than we did, the job is far more complex. I am still not sure whether the high grades required for medical school entry are necessary. The doctors produced at the London today are more academically trained and assessed more thoroughly. I am sure the three doctors I met will have a great future after the superb training they have undertaken. One does not always appreciate what good teaching is when one is relatively young.

The morning of my meeting the three doctors, I travelled from Yorkshire to Whitechapel, London, to visit what was called the London Hospital in my day. When I emerged from Whitechapel underground station, I was shocked by what faced me.

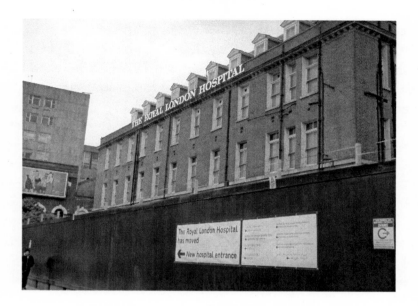

The Royal London Hospital has moved.

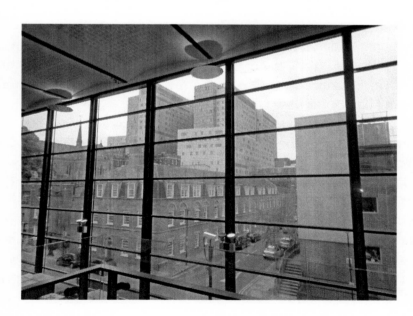

View of the new hospital from the Turner Street side of the Blizard Building.

I met Prof. Tom MacDonald, dean of research at Barts and the London School of Medicine and Dentistry. The situation with Ph.D. students and lecturers is a far cry from that of the 1970s. To become a Ph.D. student, there is an application process that can be undertaken online. A project or area of work is chosen. After shortlisting, there is a rigorous interview. Tom Macdonald told me he could tell whether an applicant would make a good researcher by 'looking into her or his eyes'. At that point, I looked away! The Ph.D. student starts with a grant for the work and a supervisor. I got the impression that translational research (translates into medical practice) would attract a grant more easily than basic research. However, the Medical Research Council is still supplying considerable funding for basic or pure research. The UK has a particularly good reputation for pure research. The University of London funded my work in physiology. There are no teaching commitments for Ph.D. students. I would not have liked that situation personally. The final viva is more rigorous than in my day, and rather than one's supervisor, the internal examiner is from the University of London with the external being from anywhere in the UK. The Ph.D. student may fail outright, have to resubmit within a specified time, or undertake further experiments under guidance. Work is periodically presented in-house. Publication of the work is encouraged so that most of the thesis has been peer reviewed before the viva.

Seventy per cent of the applications are from non-medically qualified applicants. The Ph.D. can take three or four years to complete. For the medically qualified, their NHS salary is maintained for thirty-six months.

I was surprised to hear that a significant percentage of Ph.D. students failed to write up their theses despite considerable persuasion. In the 1960s and 1970s, I never heard of anyone who embarked on a Ph.D. and who failed to submit. Professor MacDonald's bookshelves housed a dozen or more Ph.D. theses written under his supervision. He did tell me that there was no such thing as physiology any more. I never really go to the bottom of this. Bill Keatinge will be turning in his grave.

Non-clinical lecturers are required to have a Ph.D. and have undertaken two three-year periods of work in different institutions. Clinical lecturers also had to possess a Ph.D. and have worked in the NHS for five years. A clinical senior lecturer was usually given consultant status. Queen Mary College runs a course over a year or more on educational methods. All lecturers have to undertake this course, which results in a teaching qualification.

I was shown around the huge glass-sided Blizard Building, which is home for a number of hundreds of research workers.

In the Blizard Building, there is a 400-seat state-of-the-art lecture theatre and two seminar rooms that look as though they are suspended in mid air. Part of the building houses several private businesses' offices. A researcher working with business can have a share of any royalties. This was not so in my time. The invention of the ZGAT by me and Bill Keatinge and its subsequent manufacture provided the very first royalties to the London Hospital Medical College. We were one of the first researchers there to work with business.

I went for a walk around the hospital and came across buildings named after people I knew or had worked for. There was a Donniach room as well as Floyer House (the students' hostel) and the Wingate building.

I went into the GP out-of-hours drop in centre situated near the A & E department. I spoke to two of the receptionists who work there in the daytime despite the centre not opening until the evening. Patients had written down the telephone number and there was a stream of phone calls coming in all day from patients who had to be redirected. A & E used to direct cases to be seen by the GPs but this has stopped. There used to be GPs working in the A & E departments but this is no longer the situation.

The medical school and hospital have become enormous and impressive. This has involved merger with Queen Mary's and St Barts. The student intake of 400 means that not all can experience the London hospital to the full like I did. However, the experience of studying and working in this vast campus with such excellent facilities must be one of the best in the UK.

After The London I was a partner working in the Leckhampton Road Surgery in Cheltenham.

The Leckhampton Road Surgery was sold and a new building bought in the Moorend Park Road. I was invited to the opening ceremony round about 1980. Tony Mules, my senior partner, shouted across the room on my arrival—'Get out now, boy'. He was advising me to pack in general practice as it had become so awful in his eyes. The new building had a first-floor flat. The practice was kind enough to let Mary Mayo, the retired practice nurse, live there until she passed away. The flat is now an office occupied by Sue Careswell, the practice manager. She kindly spoke to me on the telephone to tell me how the practice had developed over the years.

The practice serves a population of 12,500, 2000 more than when I worked there. There are eight equity partners and also a salaried partner. Four of the partners undertook their training in London medical schools. (I can count on the fingers of both hands the number of doctors out of the 250 or so working in the Wakefield District who qualified in London). We were five partners for 10,000 patients. Two of the partners are trainers and the practice takes two trainees. The only outside job is a clinical assistantship in ear, nose, and throat surgery and this is also a specialty in the practice. The practice also undertakes endometrial biopsies (biopsies of the lining of the womb). There are five practice nurses and three health-care assistants. We had one practice nurse, Mary Mayo. There are six working in administration including two secretaries. The increase in doctors, nurses, management and administration people is an indication of the huge workload of the practice compared with my day.

There is a large conference room that is also used for teaching. It is possible, with the development of 1,000 houses in the suburb of Shurdington, that the practice moves to a site there with an even larger building.

I telephoned the practice at 191 Roehampton Road, where I worked for a few months and where the Tintners lived and had their surgery. I was put through to Carol Ward, who, amazingly, worked there when I was there. She remembered my mother who also helped out with surgeries from time to time. Carol has worked there for thirty-five years and is now a manager/receptionist. The whole of the building is a surgery. It is a main surgery with three GPs and twelve staff. There is a branch surgery in Putney. There are about 7,500 patients, but there are no longer any private patients. Gerda Tintner had a special interest in psychiatry. The practice has a psychologist undertaking some sessions.

I met Monica Smith, a half-time equity partner at my old practice. Tieve Tara Medical Centre has about 5,100 patients, roughly the same as when I retired in 2005. The practice has continued with two GP trainers (Anne Godridge and Graham Bond). There are now four GP trainees. Fortunately, the new building is large enough for each GP and trainee to have his or her own consulting room. Monica oversees third-year medical student attachments and the practice takes in two students for twenty-five weeks of the year. Russell Potts took over as practice manager when Celia Burnhope, the practice development manager, retired. In 2010, the PCT made the decision that the practice was overfunded and withdrew 20 per cent of the funding. Rosario Vega, a salaried partner, was made redundant along with Samantha McKay, a health-care assistant. I have never heard of a GP partner being made redundant. In my time we certainly were well funded. This was because of the deprived area we worked in. Rosario looked after the huge nursing home with a young disabled unit. This work was taken over by Ben Young, the newest partner. The workload has increased year on year. The partners now have to justify A & E attendances as well as referrals to consultants. There are more health-care workers coming in to see patients, and it is fortunate that there are enough consulting rooms to accommodate them. For example, there is a health worker seeing drug misusers and an in-house physiotherapy service. The doctors and nurses are following up more patients who have been treated by the hospital. There are more guidelines and pathways to follow. The service commitment of four trainees covers more than the workload of the partner who left. The partners are sure there will be a complaint leading to litigation and tend to practise somewhat defensively. That means they will admit and investigate patients more than that is strictly necessary. This is a problem when the pressure is on all GPs to admit less and refer less. Anne Godridge is the senior partner and has reduced her work commitment to four days a week from five. This is a trend with all GPs and is partly explained by their larger salaries and increased workload.

David Brown, with whom I worked as a course organiser, met me to discuss GP training. Training to become a GP had changed considerably since I was involved. In my time, Wakefield, Dewsbury, and Pontefract each had a postgraduate centre and the West Riding GPEC was responsible for about thirty GP trainees (later called registrars). In 2012, there is a superbly equipped postgraduate centre situated in the grounds of the new Pinderfields Hospital at Wakefield. Pontefract's Postgraduate Centre closed down and Dewsbury's continues. The West Riding General Practice Speciality Training Programme (formerly the GPEC) has 115 general practice specialty training registrars (GP StRs, formally called trainees) managed by 7 general practice specialty training programme directors (formerly called course organisers). These titles change with monotonous regularity. There has been a huge increase in trainees, but the number of applicants has been falling since 2010.

Recruitment of GP StRs is managed by the National Recruitment Office for General Practice Training.[24] Applications are made electronically after which shortlisting occurs using the results from two national assessments. Applicants have indicated their deanery preferences. The first assessment is a clinical problem solving test. The second assessment is a situational judgement test. If shortlisted, the candidate enters the

24   http://www.gprecruitment.org.uk/

regional selection process. This involves a written test and three simulation exercises. One of the simulation tests deals with a colleague, the others with patients. If successful, the deanery will allocate a new GP StR to a programme. This selection process started its evolution during my time at the deanery. I have not gone into any details about the assessments but wanted to demonstrate how rigorous the process has become.

GP StRs spend eighteen months in a training general practice compared with the year in my time. It has been agreed that this will be increased further.

There is a written curriculum for GP training as well as a detailed trainee trajectory. The latter is a three-year map, which describes in detail, month on month, about clinical attachments, courses, and assessments. Since 2007, for a doctor to obtain a certificate of completion of training, he or she must become a Member of the Royal College of General Practitioners (MRCGP). Becoming a member is integrated within the three-year training course. It involves an applied knowledge test, a clinical skills assessment, and a workplace-based assessment. Evidence for the latter is collected in an e-portfolio. Details of these are on the Royal College of General Practitioners' web site.[25] Throughout the three-year training, GP StRs have an educational supervisor separate from their trainer. Conversations with their supervisor can be confidential.

One of the main reasons I took the MRCGP examination in 1984 was that I had heard that in Oxfordshire it was mandatory to have this qualification in order to become a trainer. The Yorkshire Deanery introduced this rule in 1999. However, trainers at that time without this qualification were allowed to continue. As well as the MRCGP, trainers must noe also possess the Postgraduate Certificate in Primary Care Education. This can be obtained by undertaking a one—or two-year part-time course. After an initial approval visit, there is a reapproval

---

[25]   http://www.rcgp.org.uk/

assessment after a year and after that every five years (it was three in my time).

In order to become approved as a new training practice, there is a rigorous inspection of all the deanery requirements. These requirements have been updated with time and can be found on the Yorkshire and the Humber web pages.[26]

Programme directors are hard to recruit and are appointed after interview.

There is now whole-day release training. David Brown (one of the programme directors) has a surgery in Normanton with a huge training suite that can be used at the same time as the Wakefield Postgraduate Centre. Richard Adams, programme director, Dewsbury, has similar training facilities in his surgery. These superb teaching units have been part-funded by the deanery.

Gone are the Summer School and other residential seminars. Instead there are regular locality-based whole-day seminars for the programme directors and one annual seminar for a larger geographical area. I find this change truly awful as I valued learning from and teaching on these longer residential seminars fulfilling and enriching. They must have cost a lot of money to run.

There are no longer GP tutors providing education for established GPs. This is managed by the PCT, which will be abolished in 2013.

Our strategic health authority, NHS Yorkshire and the Humber, has merged with two other strategic health authorities to form NHS North of England. David Brown is the GP representative for West Yorkshire on the newly established Yorkshire and Humber Local Education and Training Board.[27] Its remit is to advise NHS North of England on all matters relating to NHS education as well as to develop a strategy

---

26   http://www.yorksandhumberdeanery.nhs.uk/
27   http://www.yorksandhumber.nhs.uk/

and business plan. These reorganisations are in preparation for the implementation of the Health and Social Care Act in April 2013.

The Yorkshire Deanery has greatly enlarged having merged with areas in South Yorkshire, Humberside, and North Lincolnshire. It is now called the Yorkshire and the Humber Postgraduate Deanery. The head office is in the building where I worked on the Leeds University Campus (Willow Terrace Road). The deanery is divided into three—North East Yorkshire and Lincolnshire, South and West Yorkshire. Each of these areas has a base with West Yorkshire housed in the headquarters. Mark Purvis was a fellow associate director in the early 2000s. He became the director of postgraduate general practice education after George Taylor left. In 2006, Adrian Dunbar is the only other person working in the deanery, who was an associate director in my time. He met me for lunch to discuss the work of the deanery today. His job title is associate postgraduate dean, and it was intended that his job embraced both general practice and hospital training. This has not happened for him. There are a couple of consultant associate deans who are managing aspects of general practice training. I am sure this is not a good thing because of the huge cultural gap between hospital and general practice, which I saw widening when I was working in the deanery. Appraisal of programme directors (course organisers) has been discontinued. All the Yorkshire GP tutors were made redundant as the PCTs took over the facilitation of GP education. I described the recruitment and assessment of trainees above. Adrian has responsibility for assessment. He works two sessions (a full day) each week, and he does very little travelling associated with the work. I travelled a lot and worked four sessions a week. Other associate directors in my time worked a greater number of sessions than four. The other areas managed by associate deans are performance and recruiting. The West Yorkshire part of the deanery manages about 300 trainees and it is to everyone's credit that most of these stay and work in Yorkshire. This is not so with the training of doctors planning to become consultants. Since I left, the deanery has put a lot of money into practice buildings to provide education facilities of a high standard. My own practice funded its own superb education suite, which I regularly rent for the meetings of the Education Support Group I manage. There are many training practices in Yorkshire with equally excellent education facilities.

Speaking to Adrian and others about the deanery, I gained the impression that it was not a happy place to work. I am sure that the relentless reorganisations contribute to this unhappiness.

The PCT's protected learning for GPs (TARGET) continues to be managed by the events manager, Anthony Nicholas. The main change is that I no longer am the education advisor and was not replaced. Instead, GPs with special interests are brought in for advice. There are GPs on the TARGET planning group. There are six afternoons when big educational events are held and six in-house general practice afternoon learning times. Little has changed.

The QOF now takes in more NICE guidance into targets. Kevin Duggan left the PCT to work as a practice manager in Pontefract. He used to be the person dealing with pedantic queries from practice managers and now he is making the enquiries himself! The new QOF lead, Linda Reynolds, worked with Kevin. She easily took over the reins. In 2011/12, the payment for one QOF point was £130.51. The total paid to a practice is weighted according to the number of patients. It is still a very significant amount of money for a practice. That year the PCT paid out well over seven million pounds to practices working in the Wakefield District. There is no longer an inspection of each practice. This has been reduced to two random visits. There is a GP, a practice manager, a layperson, and a PCT manager in the inspection team. Practices submit evidence of their claims to claim the points. This evidence is examined by a panel consisting of a GP, a layperson, a practice manager, the QOF lead, and Karen Tooley (performance improvement manager). The new system is not a national one but is used by the three PCTs that merged in 2010 to become what is known as a cluster. The advantage of the panel is that procedures etc. can be looked at in detail and poor evidence submitted can be discussed more openly than that during an inspection.

Alison Evans, who works as a permanent locum GP, took over my job as appraisal lead for the PCT, NHS Wakefield District. She is not the Alison Evans who worked with me at the Deanery. She met me in April 2012 to explain the changes that have occurred.

In March 2012, the coalition government announced that revalidation would start. At long last! Revalidation of each GP and locum is repeated every five years. It has been estimated that about 4 per cent might not be revalidated but allowed to be assessed again after a six-month improvement plan. Most think that a significant number of older GPs will retire now, not wishing the hassle of revalidation. In 2012, only GPs in management and education roles will be revalidated. This is about 10 per cent of the GP workforce. One of the objects of revalidation is to identify poor performance. One suspects that this first year is a pilot and that it is very unlikely indeed that any of this 10 per cent will not be revalidated.

The person who makes the decision as to whether or not to revalidate a GP is the responsible officer. He or she has to judge the supporting information supplied by the GP. Responsible officers are receiving training to ensure that the decisions made are for the same reasons nationwide. The PCT keeps a record of all GPs who are allowed to practise in the trust's area. This is called the performers' list. The PCT has the power to suspend or remove a GP from the list thus preventing him practising. In 2010, the year I retired, the number on the performers' list was about 250. There has been a significant increase in part-time salaried GPs and the list now numbers 300. In the second year of revalidation, the responsible officer will have to spend very significant time reading supporting information.

For each of the five years before revalidation, supporting information has to be collated by the GP. This includes an appraisal with PDPs; two significant events audits that must include anything serious; a patient and colleague survey; fifty learning credits; a review of complaints. Once in every five years a full-cycle clinical audit to be performed and written up. A statement will be submitted by the GP's appraiser. This statement could be regarded as vitally important by a busy overworked responsible officer.

A learning credit is one hour of education accompanied by reflective notes. In Chapter 9, I described the situation of accreditation in 1992. For that, a GP had to simply attend thirty hours of education each year without having to pay much attention. In 2012, it is fifty hours with a few notes made. I hope that there is a demand by appraisers and responsible officers for a high standard of reflective notes. In 2010, extra credits were proposed for quality reflection but this was watered down.

Recruitment of new appraisers to the Wakefield scheme is a problem. In 2012, there are fifteen appraisers, two less than that of 2010, with fifty more GPs to appraise. The reason for the difficulty recruiting is the hugely increased workload of the GPs. Every appraiser I have ever encountered found the work fascinating, fulfilling and very time-consuming.

Alison Evans has continued to run a bimonthly appraiser support group, but the talk in 2012 is mainly about revalidation. There has been some top-up training for appraisers.

Chapter 11 has a description of the excellent Internet facility for recording appraisal information and attaching supporting documents—the NHS Appraisal Toolkit. This closed down in March 2012. At that time there were twelve toolkits available, and this has resulted in considerable uncertainty. Some of these toolkits have been created by IT-savvy GPs and are free. Others have a cost. There is a revalidation ready toolkit that the PCT will fund until December 2012. The Royal College of General Practitioners have a revalidation toolkit, which is free to members but might cost £1,500 to non-members.

In April 2013, the PCTs will be abolished. The new Health and Social Care Act involves a major reorganisation of the NHS. Clinical Commissioning Groups (CCG) were set up in 2011 and these will have a huge financial budget in order to manage the NHS locally. These groups are managed by GPs. The group also has one or two nurses and hospital consultants as members. At the same time, in preparation for April 2013, PCTs have merged into clusters. Wakefield merged with Calderdale and Kirklees PCTs. There is uncertainty about how revalidation and appraisals will be managed in the future

The Health and Social Care Act was eventually given royal assent in March 2012. It had a very difficult passage through each of the houses of parliament. I objected to this bill vehemently and sent evidence to parliament's scrutiny committee. We have all known for a long time that the act will abolish the PCTs. The budget for the NHS in the Wakefield District will be devolved to a Clinical Commissioning Group of GPs (CCG). The fear is that private companies will take more and more of the NHS work. Most GPs are not in the slightest interested in yet another major reorganisation of the NHS. In my opinion, the CCG has no idea of the detailed work that the PCT has undertaken over the years. Many in the PCT have already left for new jobs, retired or been made redundant. There were 26 made redundant in 2010/11 at a cost of £1,196,698. (These facts were obtained by a Freedom of Information request by me in July 2012). The skills pool has been severely depleted. There will be a Commissioning Support Services body established. It will employ people from the abolished PCT to carry things forward. At the time of writing, no one I have met knows how the NHS will develop in the Wakefield area. Indeed, no one really knows how the NHS will develop in England over the next few years.

After reading this book, I wonder how people will answer these questions. Why do students have to achieve such high A-level grades to gain entry to medical school? Is the undergraduate medical education of a higher quality now than in the 1960s? Is an integrated B.Sc. at UCL a better experience than specialising for eighteen months on anatomy, physiology, biochemistry, or pharmacology? How does studying as a clinical student compare? Is the Ph.D. student better supported these days and undertaking research freely? Should a lecturer be required to have Ph.D.? Is it a good thing that lecturers have to learn about educational methods? Has vocational training improved over the years such that patients are consulting with better and better GPs? Has computerisation of medical records helped with management of diseases? Does the postgraduate education of GPs mean that most are up to date? Are GPs better communicators than those in the past? Will revalidation prevent another Harold Shipman? Finally, will the NHS survive the radical changes introduced in 2012?

INDEX

A

Adams, Dawn   119
Adams, Richard   234
ADH (antidiuretic hormone)   107
Agawala, Jyoti   145
Agnes (Sam's wife)   25-7
Alba-Mendez, Paula   210
Alison (Angela and John's daughter)   27
amphetamine   38, 153
Amy (Caroline's daughter)   129
Andrew (Gerry and Johnny's son)   15
Angela (Sam and Agnes's daughter)   25, 27
Ann (Colin Teasdale's wife)   56, 73
Annette (Bill Keatinge's wife)   105
Anthony, Dick   111
Armstrong, Lynn   142, 146
Armstrong-James, Mike   93
Arnett, Tim   221
Ash, Danny   72
Asian flu epidemic   22
Atchamah, Natasha   11, 223
Aunty Gladys   75
Averil (Stephen's wife)   98

B

Bahrami, Jamie   47, 158, 160, 172, 174, 180-1, 183-7, 190, 193-5, 197
Bailey and Love (Mann)   70
Baker, Richard   119
Baker, Sarah   135, 145
Balint, Michael   122
Balint Society   122
Barbara (Steve Shalet's wife)   73
Barbier, Brian   52
barbiturate   38
Barker, Mark   140
Barker, Philip   216
Barnado, Thomas   58
Barnett, Tony   100
Barron, Julie   152
Barrowman, Jim   92, 94
Bazaz, Mohan   139, 141-2, 145
Bearsted Lecture Theatre   66
Beckmann thermometer   96-7
Belk, Jeremy   176
Belton, Andrew   173
Bert (Maureen's husband)   18
Bibby, John   171-2, 197, 209

T

U

V

Lightning Source UK Ltd.
Milton Keynes UK
UKOW040329290912

199836UK00001B/37/P